Genitourinary Ultrasound I

Guest Editors

PAUL S. SIDHU, MBBS, MRCP, FRCR
MUKUND JOSHI, MD

ULTRASOUND CLINICS

www.ultrasound.theclinics.com

July 2010 • Volume 5 • Number 3

SAUNDERS an imprint of ELSEVIER, Inc.

W.B. SAUNDERS COMPANY
A Division of Elsevier Inc.

1600 John F. Kennedy Boulevard • Suite 1800 • Philadelphia, Pennsylvania 19103-2899

http://www.theclinics.com

ULTRASOUND CLINICS Volume 5, Number 3
July 2010 ISSN 1556-858X, ISBN-13: 978-1-4377-2597-1

Editor: Barton Dudlick

Ultrasound Clinics (ISSN 1556-858X) is published quarterly by W.B. Saunders, 360 Park Avenue South, New York, NY 10010-1710. Months of publication are January, April, July, and October. Business and editorial offices: 1600 John F. Kennedy Boulevard, Suite 1800, Philadelphia, Pennsylvania 19103-2899. Accounting and circulation offices: 6277 Sea Harbor Drive, Orlando, FL 32887-4800. Periodicals postage paid at New York, NY, and additional mailing offices. Subscription prices are $204 per year for (US individuals), $279 per year for (US institutions), $102 per year for (US students and residents), $232 per year for (Canadian individuals), $312 per year for (Canadian institutions), $247 per year for (international individuals), $312 per year for (international institutions), and $123 per year for (Canadian and foreign students/residents). To receive student/resident rate, orders must be accompanied by name of affiliated institution, date of term, and the signature of program/residency coordinator on institution letterhead. Orders will be billed at individual rate until proof of status is received. Foreign air speed delivery is included in all Clinics subscription prices. All prices are subject to change without notice. **POSTMASTER:** Send address changes to *Ultrasound Clinics*, Elsevier Health Sciences Division, Subscription Customer Service, 3251 Riverport Lane, Maryland Heights, MO 63043. **Customer Service (orders, claims, online, change of address): Telephone: 1-800-654-2452 (U.S. and Canada); 314-447-8871 (outside U.S. and Canada). Fax: 314-447-8029. E-mail: journalscustomerservice-usa@elsevier.com (for print support); journalsonlinesupport-usa@elsevier.com (for online support).**

Reprints: For copies of 100 or more, of articles in this publication, please contact the Commercial Reprints Department, Elsevier Inc., 360 Park Avenue South, New York, NY 10010-1710. Tel.: (+1) 212-633-3812; Fax: (+1) 212-462-1935; E-mail: reprints@elsevier.com.

Printed and bound by CPI Group (UK) Ltd, Croydon, CR0 4YY

Transferred to Digital Print 2012

Contributors

CONSULTING EDITOR

VIKRAM S. DOGRA, MD
Professor of Radiology, Urology, and
Biomedical Engineering, Director of Ultrasound
and Associate Chair for Education and
Research, Department of Imaging Sciences,
University of Rochester School of Medicine
and Dentistry, Rochester, New York

GUEST EDITORS

PAUL S. SIDHU, MBBS, MRCP, FRCR
Consultant Radiologist and Senior Lecturer,
Department of Diagnostic Radiology,
King's College Hospital, Denmark Hill,
London, United Kingdom

MUKUND JOSHI, MD
Dr Joshi's Imaging Clinic, Mumbai,
Maharashtra, India

AUTHORS

PIYUSH K. AGARWAL, MD
Department of Urology, Case Western
Reserve University School of Medicine
and University Hospitals of Cleveland,
Cleveland, Ohio

DONALD R. BODNER, MD
Department of Urology, Case Western
Reserve University School of Medicine
and University Hospitals of Cleveland,
Cleveland, Ohio

ANJUMARA BORA, DMRE, DNB
Clinical Assistant, Department of Ultrasound,
Dr Balabhai Nanavati Hospital and Research
Center, Mumbai, Maharashtra, India

VIKRAM S. DOGRA, MD
Professor of Radiology, Urology, and
Biomedical Engineering, Director of Ultrasound
and Associate Chair for Education and
Research, Department of Imaging Sciences,
University of Rochester School of Medicine
and Dentistry, Rochester, New York

DANIEL T. GINAT, MD, MS
Department of Imaging Sciences,
University of Rochester Medical Center,
Rochester, New York

SUDHEER GOKHALE, MD, FICR, FICMU
Honorary Consultant, Department of
Imaging Sciences, Choithram Hospital
and Research Centre, Indore,
Madhya Pradesh, India

ALKA S. KARNIK, MD
Consultant Radiologist and Head of
Department of Ultrasound, Dr Balabhai
Nanavati Hospital and Research Center,
Mumbai, Maharashtra, India

ANEETA PARTHIPUN, MBBS, FRCR
Radiology Department, St George's Hospital,
London, United Kingdom

JAMES PILCHER, MBBS, MSc, MRCP, FRCR
Radiology Department, St George's Hospital,
London, United Kingdom

WAEL E.A. SAAD, MD
Department of Radiology,
University of Virginia Health System,
Charlottesville, Virginia

S. BOOPATHY VIJAYARAGHAVAN, MD, DMRD
Consultant Diagnostic Radiologist, Sonoscan:
Ultrasonic Scan Centre, RS Puram,
Coimbatore, Tamil Nadu, India

SRINIVAS VOURGANTI, MD
Department of Urology, Case Western Reserve
University School of Medicine, University
Hospitals of Cleveland, Cleveland, Ohio

Contents

Doppler Ultrasonography in Renovascular Hypertension   337

Sudheer Gokhale

> Color Doppler ultrasonography is an excellent screening modality for renovascular hypertension (RVH). The technique is one of the most challenging ultrasound examinations; nevertheless, with expertise and skill, it is possible to perform a technically acceptable examination in most patients. This article will highlight this technique's use in patients with RVH.

Ultrasonographic Evaluation of Renal Infections   355

Srinivas Vourganti, Piyush K. Agarwal, Donald R. Bodner, and Vikram S. Dogra

> Renal sonography can be easily performed and provides valuable information concerning the underlying disease process, helping to decide appropriate management. This article reviews the important renal infections, such as pyelonephritis, emphysematous pyelonephritis, renal abscess, hydatid disease, renal tuberculosis, pyonephrosis, and human immunodeficiency virus–associated nephropathy.

Ultrasonography of Genitourinary Tuberculosis   367

S. Boopathy Vijayaraghavan

> Genitourinary tuberculosis is the second most common form of extrapulmonary tuberculosis after lymph node involvement and may account for between 30% and 41% of nonpulmonary cases. The kidney is usually the primary organ infected in urinary disease, and other parts of the urinary tract become involved by direct extension. The epididymis in men and the fallopian tubes in women are the primary sites of genital infection. Tuberculosis of the male and female genital tracts and its ultrasonographic features are discussed in this article.

Renal Transplant Assessment: Sonographic Imaging   379

Aneeta Parthipun and James Pilcher

> Renal transplant graft survival rates have improved markedly in the past 30 years because of improvements in operative techniques, tissue typing, and immunosuppressive agents. This article outlines the approach to transplant ultrasonography and reviews its role in the diagnosis and management of various recognized complications, both early and late in the graft's life span. Although relatively accurate in diagnosing vascular complications, fluid collections, urological complications, and late-onset diseases of the graft, ultrasonography still has limited specificity in the early stages of delayed graft function, often requiring transplant biopsy to make the distinction. Recently developed techniques are discussed including using contrast agents to obtain functional information about the transplant, which may avoid the need for some biopsies in the future.

Ultrasound-Guided Therapeutic Urological Interventions   401

Daniel T. Ginat and Wael E.A. Saad

> Interventional uroradiology is a well-established discipline that offers minimal-invasive treatment options for a wide spectrum of urinary system conditions.

Many interventional uroradiology procedures are amenable to ultrasound guidance, either alone or in combination with other modalities, such as fluoroscopy and computed tomography. In this article, indications, techniques, and outcomes of ultrasound-guided nephrostomy, cyst aspiration, sclerotherapy, and suprapubic catheterization are reviewed and illustrated.

Antenatal ultrasonography is an excellent modality that can diagnose most abnormalities of the fetal genitorurinary tract. The typical findings of various abnormalities help in accurate prenatal diagnosis. Reduced amniotic fluid is the first clue to compromised fetal renal function. With known urinary obstruction, serial follow-up ultrasonography to monitor increasing hydronephrosis and developing post obstructive dysplasia helps in obstetric and neonatal management. MR imaging gives valuable information in difficult cases, especially when there is gross oligohydramnios and poor resolution on the ultrasonography examination.

Ultrasound Clinics

THE CLINICS ARE NOW AVAILABLE ONLINE!

Access your subscription at:
www.theclinics.com

GOAL STATEMENT

The goal of the *Ultrasound Clinics* is to keep practicing radiologists and radiology residents up to date with current clinical practice in ultrasound by providing timely articles reviewing the state of the art in patient care.

ACCREDITATION

The *Ultrasound Clinics* is planned and implemented in accordance with the Essential Areas and Policies of the Accreditation Council for Continuing Medical Education (ACCME) through the joint sponsorship of the University of Virginia School of Medicine and Elsevier. The University of Virginia School of Medicine is accredited by the ACCME to provide continuing medical education for physicians.

The University of Virginia School of Medicine designates this educational activity for a maximum of 15 *AMA PRA Category 1 Credits*™ for each issue, 60 credits per year. Physicians should only claim credit commensurate with the extent of their participation in the activity.

The American Medical Association has determined that physicians not licensed in the US who participate in this CME activity are eligible for a maximum of 15 **AMA PRA Category 1 Credits**™ for each issue, 60 credits per year.

Credit can be earned by reading the text material, taking the CME examination online at http://www.theclinics.com/home/cme, and completing the evaluation. After taking the test, you will be required to review any and all incorrect answers. Following completion of the test and evaluation, your credit will be awarded and you may print your certificate.

FACULTY DISCLOSURE/CONFLICT OF INTEREST

The University of Virginia School of Medicine, as an ACCME accredited provider, endorses and strives to comply with the Accreditation Council for Continuing Medical Education (ACCME) Standards of Commercial Support, Commonwealth of Virginia statutes, University of Virginia policies and procedures, and associated federal and private regulations and guidelines on the need for disclosure and monitoring of proprietary and financial interests that may affect the scientific integrity and balance of content delivered in continuing medical education activities under our auspices.

The University of Virginia School of Medicine requires that all CME activities accredited through this institution be developed independently and be scientifically rigorous, balanced and objective in the presentation/discussion of its content, theories and practices.

All authors/editors participating in an accredited CME activity are expected to disclose to the readers relevant financial relationships with commercial entities occurring within the past 12 months (such as grants or research support, employee, consultant, stock holder, member of speakers bureau, etc.). The University of Virginia School of Medicine will employ appropriate mechanisms to resolve potential conflicts of interest to maintain the standards of fair and balanced education to the reader. Questions about specific strategies can be directed to the Office of Continuing Medical Education, University of Virginia School of Medicine, Charlottesville, Virginia.

The faculty and staff of the University of Virginia Office of Continuing Medical Education have no financial affiliations to disclose.

The authors/editors listed below have identified no professional or financial affiliations for themselves or their spouse/partner:
Matthew J. Bassignani, MD (Test Author); Anjumara Bora, DMRE, DNB; Vikram S. Dogra, MD (Consulting Editor); Barton Dudlick, (Acquisitions Editor); Daniel T. Ginat, MD, MS; Sudheer Gokhale, MD, FICR, FICMU; Mukund Joshi, MD (Guest Editor); Alka S. Karnik, MD; Aneeta Parthipun, MBBS, FRCR; James Pilcher, MBBS, MSc, MRCP, FRCR; Wael E. A. Saad, MD, MS; S. Boopathy Vijayaraghavan, MD, DMRD; and Srinivas Vourganti, MD.

The authors/editors listed below have identified the following professional or financial affiliations for themselves or their spouse/partner:
Piyush K. Agarwal, MD's spouse is employed by Astellas Pharmaceuticals; is on the Speakers' Bureau for Endo Pharmaceuticals.
Donald R. Bodner, MD owns stock in Fortec Litho and Medtronic.
Paul S. Sidhu, MBBS, MRCP, FRCR (Guest Editor) is on the Speakers' Bureau for Bracco (SpA, Milan), Hitachi Japan, and Siemens AG Germany.

Disclosure of Discussion of Non-FDA Approved Uses for Pharmaceutical Products and/or Medical Devices.

The University of Virginia School of Medicine, as an ACCME provider, requires that all faculty presenters identify and disclose any off-label uses for pharmaceutical and medical device products. The University of Virginia School of Medicine recommends that each physician fully review all the available data on new products or procedures prior to clinical use.

TO ENROLL

To enroll in the Ultrasound Clinics Continuing Medical Education program, call customer service at 1-800-654-2452 or visit us online at http://www.theclinics.com/home/cme. The CME program is available to subscribers for an additional fee of $196.00.

Preface
Genitourinary Ultrasound

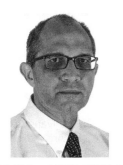
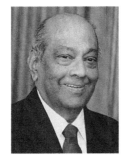

Paul S. Sidhu, MBBS, MRCP, FRCR   Mukund Joshi, MD
Guest Editors

This edition of the *Ultrasound Clinics* differs from any preceding issues from the series in one important aspect: we have assembled an array of experts from around the world in order to present the reader with a global and expert view of genitourinary sonography.

Imaging of the genitourinary tract presents many challenges with myriad disease processes presenting with symptoms attributable to the genitourinary system. Sonography remains the first-line imaging procedure and, in many instances, in the child and the neonate, the only imaging modality used. Technical factors related to transducer capabilities, increasing sophistication of computing processing, and the advent of digital imaging have all contributed to a vast improvement in sonographic imaging over the last decade, culminating in the production of exquisite images of diagnostic value. The "discovery" of contrast media that can be used in sonography has revolutionized imaging of the kidneys and is now an accepted technique in many countries where the product is licensed for use (not in the US yet!). Indeed in the assessment of complex renal cysts and vascular infarction, the transplant kidney may well be regarded as the "gold standard" in the future. Two articles address the use of contrast media in renal disease in the native and transplant kidney.

Imaging the unborn fetus is never easy, and making a confident interpretation of the many appearances is a great skill to attain. Management is greatly influenced by the findings, and a comprehensive review details the use of sonography in the fetal genitourinary tract. Pediatric diseases of the genitourinary tract are very varied and essentially different from that in the adult, with the renal mass presenting a challenge. A clear understanding is important, with a comprehensive and well-illustrated article addressing this aspect.

In the adult patient, renal infections are often problematic, nearly always in the Western world attributable to a bacterial infection. Not so on a worldwide context were tuberculosis affects the entire genitourinary tract, producing characteristic sonographic features. These two aspects are dealt with in two articles giving a perspective of infectious diseases affecting the kidneys. Remember that tuberculosis is on its way back in many countries where the disease had all but been eradicated.

Hypertension remains a worldwide problem with severe long-term consequences for the health budget of a country if allowed to cause end-organ damage; it is a "silent" disease. Renal causes are often treatable, and a cost-effective test for this is available with the use of sonography. An article comprehensively covers the diagnosis and pitfalls and reviews the available evidence for the use of sonography to image renal hypertension.

There is often a paucity of information in the literature with regards to male health, which is addressed by articles on the prostate and testis, with a third article on the bladder also presented for good measure. Sonography is the first-line imaging procedure in all three anatomical areas

Ultrasound Clin 5 (2010) ix–x
doi:10.1016/j.cult.2010.09.001

and often provides a comprehensive view of the abnormalities commonly afflicting these areas. The testis is especially suited to sonography with recourse to other imaging rarely necessary.

Last, minimally invasive techniques are deployed more frequently than ever before to treat diseases of the genitourinary tract, and these procedures are invariably guided by sonography. The skill required to guide intervention by sonography is immense, but often underappreciated by clinical colleagues. An article addresses the common procedures in a very practical manner.

It is with great pleasure that we recommend this book to you, with a wide array of expert reviews from around the world detailing advances and practical aspects and comprehensively illustrating the many and varied monographic appearances of common, unusual, and rare manifestations of genitourinary disease. We hope you enjoy and benefit from the book.

Paul S. Sidhu, MBBS, MRCP, FRCR
Department of Radiology
King's College Hospital
Denmark Hill
London SE5 9RS, UK

Mukund Joshi, MD
Dr Joshi's Imaging Clinic
809 Harjivandas Estate
Dr Ambedkar Road
Dadar East, Mumbai 400014, Maharashtra, India

E-mail addresses:
paulsidhu@btinternet.com (P.S. Sidhu)
drmukundjoshi@gmail.com (M. Joshi)

Doppler Ultrasonography in Renovascular Hypertension

Sudheer Gokhale, MD, FICR, FICMU*

KEYWORDS

- Renovascular Hypertension • Doppler
- Renal artery stenosis

Renovascular hypertension (RVH) occurs when blood pressure rises as a consequence of renal ischemia. Goldblatt, in his renowned experiment in 1934, demonstrated that occlusion of the renal artery creates ischemia, which triggers the release of renin and causes secondary hypertension.[1] RVH resulting from renal artery stenosis is a potentially curable form of secondary hypertension. The kidney is both the culprit and the victim; often there is a vicious cycle between renovascular disease, which causes hypertension, which in turn causes more renal damage. The earlier one can detect this situation, the less likely it is that permanent and irreversible renal damage occurs.

CLINICAL BACKGROUND

Hypertension is a primary phenomenon in most patients in whom no cause is found, termed essential hypertension, accounting for 95% to 99% of the patients. Secondary hypertension affects a small group, estimated to affect between 1% and 5% of all hypertensive patients. Hypertension secondary to renal artery stenosis affects an even smaller portion, constituting between 1% and 2% of patients[2,3] in some series but up to 2% to 5% of patients in another more recent series.[4] This incidence is changing for two reasons; an aging population will be susceptible to atherosclerotic renal disease, and advancement in technology has improved detection rates of renal artery stenosis.

RVH is defined as a chronic increase in blood pressure as a consequence of renal artery stenosis. Two distinct age groups are more commonly affected.[5] The pediatric and young adult group with hypertension secondary to a renovascular cause often remain undetected and present late with complications including encephalopathy, intracranial hemorrhage, or hypertensive cardiomyopathy. Hypertension secondary to a renovascular cause is more common in this group than in adults. Several studies indicate an incidence of up to 10% in an unselected pediatric population.[6,7] The second group where hypertension secondary to a renovascular cause occurs is the elderly, where there is a high prevalence of atherosclerosis. As essential hypertension is quite common in this age group, the suspicion of a renovascular cause is often based on change in the behavior of blood pressure or onset of unexplained renal failure.[8] Renovascular disease and essential hypertension may coexist, and detection of renal artery disease does not always establish the diagnosis of RVH in this group of patients. This may necessitate a trial by a revascularization procedure; reduction in blood pressure implies a caue—effect relationship.[9,10]

It is not possible to image all patients with hypertension; the detection rates will be less than 1% and irrational in terms of cost-effectiveness. An awareness of the manner in which patients with RVH present helps in the selection of patients appropriate for diagnostic imaging. Therefore it makes good judgment to screen only those

Department of Imaging Sciences, Choithram Hospital and Research Centre, Indore, India
* Ultrasonography Clinic, 569 MG Road, Indore 452001, Madhya Pradesh, India.
E-mail address: sudheergokhale@hotmail.com

Ultrasound Clin 5 (2010) 337–353
doi:10.1016/j.cult.2010.07.002

patients who are considered to be at high risk for RVH. With a preselection protocol adhered to, the yield for a renovascular cause is as high as 15% to 32%.[5,11–13] The generally accepted criteria for preselection of patients are as follows

Accelerated hypertension

Hypertension not responding to optimal medical treatment

Young hypertensive (age <20 years)

Known hypertensive with recent, unexplained deterioration in renal function

Significant renal size difference in patients who have developed recent hypertension

Development of renal failure with angiotensin converting enzyme (ACE) inhibitors

Recurrent or flash pulmonary edema

Hypertensive patients with a clear abdominal bruit (an innocent bruit is common in younger individuals).

PATHOPHYSIOLOGY

Renal ischemia triggers an increase in secretion of renin by the juxtaglomerular apparatus of the kidney. Renin release accelerates conversion of angiotensinogen, a hormone secreted by the liver, to angiotensin 1. A further process undertaken by an enzyme, the ACE, converts angiotensin 1 into angiotensin 2, which in turn stimulates production of aldosterone. Angiotensin 2 also causes vaso-constriction in the afferent and efferent arterioles. The effect on efferent arterioles is much more significant, thereby resulting in a reduction in glomerular filtration rate (GFR). Aldosterone ulti-mately causes retention of water and sodium. In health, any sudden hypotension will trigger the re-nin–angiotensin cascade to produce efferent vasoconstriction, resulting in increased glomerular hydraulic pressure to maintain the glomerular filtration rate. In an ischemic kidney, the afferent blood flow is reduced. The glomerular filtration then is maintained by the angiotensin 2-mediated efferent vasoconstriction. Patients who are receiving ACE inhibitors lack this efferent vaso-constriction response and cannot maintain GFR with reduction in renal blood flow to the ischemic kidney. Hence in patients with bilateral renal artery stenosis or in patients with renal artery stenosis of a single kidney, ACE inhibitors may cause deterio-ration of renal function. Cessation of administra-tion of ACE inhibitors will reverse the renal dysfunction in these patients.

IMAGING OF RENAL ARTERY STENOSIS

Angiography is the established gold standard for imaging of the renal arteries. Angiography is invasive and associated with an inherent morbidity due to the procedure: vessel wall dissection, pla-que embolization, hemorrhage, infection, or due to the drugs used causing nephrotoxicity and allergic reactions. Computed tomography (CT) and magnetic resonance angiography (MRA) are other alternatives. Both imaging procedures are excellent at depicting the anatomic stenosis but do not provide any physiologic information of the consequence of stenosis. The contrast agents used during CT and MRA have nephrotoxic effects, which may be detrimental to the renal function of the individual, and they cannot be ignored. Color ultrasonography and spectral Doppler ultrasonography are noninvasive and safe providing anatomic as well as physiologic information. Ultrasonography, however, is underu-tilized for assessing renal artery stenosis, partly because of inherent difficulty in performing the examination and a high degree of operator dependence.

Doppler ultrasonography has been in use for screening of patients thought to have an under-lying renal arterial cause for hypertension for several years. One of the early investigations using ultrasonography for the assessment of renal artery stenosis used a renal artery peak systolic velocity (PSV) cut-off of 100 cm/s, with a sensitivity of 89%, to establish the presence of a significant stenosis of a renal artery.[14] Further appraisal, using the same velocity criteria, reported a sensitivity of 91% and specificity of 95% for the presence of a significant renal artery stenosis.[15] Using renal artery to aortic velocity ratio of greater than 3.5 to diagnose greater than 60% stenosis, Taylor and colleagues[16] found an overall accuracy of 93%. Other studies targeting the main renal artery PSV reported success rates of 65% to 80% for as-sessing the artery, with a sensitivity of 79% to 91% and specificity of 73% to 93% for diagnosing a renal artery stenosis.[16–18]

The targeting of the main renal artery remained problematic in these early investigations, without the benefit of technical improvements seen today. In an attempt to overcome limitations of the tech-nique of directly imaging the main renal artery, Handa and colleagues[19] described the use of in-trarenal Doppler criteria to detect a poststenotic phenomenon, the tardus–parvus spectral wave-form with an accuracy of 95%. Since then, several studies have used intrarenal Doppler criteria for detection of renal artery stenosis with success.[12,20,21] Following this initial period of enthusiasm, there was a phase when it was felt that Doppler ultrasonography failed as a screening examination due to technical difficulties where the proximal aspect of renal arteries remained nonvisualized in several patients. Subsequent studies failed to confirm earlier results, reporting poor sensitivity and accuracy of Doppler ultrasonography in detecting renal artery stenosis, mainly on account of the large number of technically inadequate examinations in these studies.[22,23]

Ultrasound machine technology improvement, and operator experience has advanced consistently over the last decade. With evolution of the dual-access practice of targeting the intrarenal arteries along with the main renal arteries, there has been a significant reduction in failed procedures and a significant improvement in overall accuracy of the technique.[24] In the author's experience, the procedural failure rate is less than 5%. Other authors report similar success rates; Zeller and colleagues[25] reported a success rate 90%, and Radermacher and colleagues[24] reported a procedure success rate of 100%. Furthermore, with the high success rate of the technical aspects of the procedure, the overall accuracy of Doppler ultrasonography as a screening test for renal artery stenosis has improved significantly. Zeller and colleagues[25] reported a sensitivity of 90% and specificity of 97%; Voiculescu and colleagues[26] reported sensitivity and specificity of 96% and 89%, and Radermacher and colleagues[24] reported a sensitivity of 96.8% and specificity of 98%.

TECHNIQUE

With the new technical advances both with the transducers and image processing, images of good quality may be achieved even in obese patients. Bowel gas is the major deterrent for an optimal examination, and it is not overcome with new technology. Although patients need not fast for the examination, small volumes of nonaerated fluid are permitted. An antiflatulent and laxative the day before the examination may help or even encouragement to take a long walk on the day of the examination. The examination should include interrogation of the kidneys and suprarenal areas. A complete anatomic examination for renal size and morphology to look for evidence of renal parenchymal disease is part of the renovascular Doppler ultrasonographic study. Particular attention should be paid to assess any differential thickness changes in different parts of each kidney, as this may be the only evidence of a segmental artery stenosis or occlusion. Examination of the suprarenal region for any abnormality of the adrenal glands to warrant further investigation for a pheochromocytoma is important. The abdominal aorta, the main renal arteries, and the intrarenal segmental or interlobar arteries are the main targets of the Doppler ultrasonographic examination. The aorta can be accessed from the anterior or anterolateral approach. The caliber of the aorta should be recorded in upper, middle and lower parts. Aortic walls should be examined for plaques and any narrowing of the lumen. From the anterior approach, aortic flow is almost perpendicular to the angle of insonation. A toe-and-heel maneuvering of the probe is useful to get good color signals, also aiding in obtaining optimal Doppler angles, so that measurement of peak systolic velocities is as accurate as possible.

The right renal artery (RRA) arises from the lateral or anterolateral aspect of the abdominal aorta, just distal to the origin of the superior mesenteric artery. It then runs posteriorly toward the inferior vena cava (IVC). In most of its course, the RRA runs perpendicular to the ultrasound beam, posing a technical challenge to create good Doppler vascular flow signals. On the other hand, this is an advantage for gray scale imaging, and the artery usually is well seen. In practice, sometimes it is difficult on an anterior approach to record good color Doppler images. It may be difficult to visualize the boundary of the RRA, as the color Doppler flow in IVC and RRA, are in the same direction and in the same color. It may be better to localize the RRA for the placement of the pulse—wave spectral Doppler sample gate, without the addition of color flow, on the gray scale images. While accessing the arteries from an anterior approach, the authors find it useful to tilt the ultrasound transducer, slightly lateral on the side examined, to obtain a better angle for the Doppler measurements. Even in obese patients, it is often not difficult to examine the distal aspect of the RRA from the anterolateral approach, using the liver as an acoustic window (**Fig. 1**). The left renal artery (LRA) originates from the lateral or posterolateral aspect of the abdominal aorta. The origin is usually just superior to the origin of the RRA. The LRA then runs laterally, posterior to the left renal vein and anterior to the psoas muscle. The distal aspect of LRA is more difficult to visualize, and can usually be viewed from the left flank, using the left kidney as an acoustic window by placing the patient in a right decubitus position (**Fig. 2**). Uncommonly, an oblique coronal approach might be needed to look for the origin of the renal arteries. The patient is placed in a partial decubitus position, and the examination is performed in an oblique coronal plane. In this view, both renal arteries are usually visible, curving out proximal and distal to the aorta. This has been termed the banana peel view (**Fig. 3**).

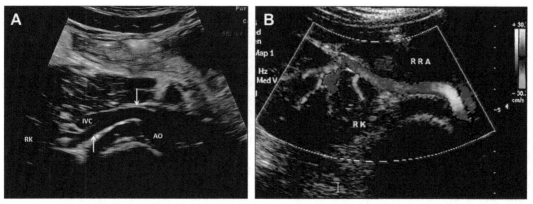

Fig. 1. Transverse images of the right renal artery (RRA). (*A*) Anterior approach, axial gray scale image of RRA *(arrows)* arising from right anterolateral aspect of aorta (AO). The RRA runs posterior to the inferior vena cava (IVC) to the right kidney (RK). (*B*) Transverse color Doppler image from anterolateral approach depicts the entire length of the RRA.

Color Doppler imaging and spectral Doppler imaging are the mainstays of the renal artery examination. Color Doppler imaging provides the mapping of renal arteries and a bird's eye view of the flow. The color gain setting should be set at highest, just below where noise appears. Pulse repetition frequency and filter settings should be adjusted according to the flow velocities in the vessel, high enough to cut off bleeding from veins, but low enough to produce aliasing at the site of stenosis. Spectral Doppler analysis is performed in the main renal arteries, ideally at every 1 cm to 2 cm along the length of the artery. If that is not technically feasible, then it should be performed at least in the proximal, middle and distal segments (**Fig. 4**). Peak Systolic velocity is recorded in the renal artery and aorta and a renal–aortic ratio (RAR) is calculated. In obese patients, color flow mapping of renal arteries may not yield a good image of the renal arteries, but as the diagnosis of stenosis in the renal arteries is solely based on analyses of spectral data, it is more important to obtain good spectral Doppler samples than color images. Therefore more attention needs to be directed toward accurate placement of sample volume gate and accurate correction of the Doppler angle.

The intrarenal arteries are approached readily from the flanks. The patient may lie supine or preferably in the decubitus position. The renal arteries and veins pass through the renal hilum in to the renal sinus space. The arteries divide into anterior and posterior branches; these in turn give off segmental, interlobar and arcuate branches. As

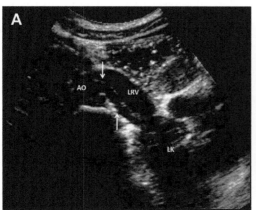
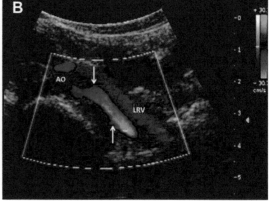

Fig. 2. Transverse images of the left renal artery (LRA). (*A*) Transverse gray scale image of the LRA *(arrows)* arising from the lateral aspect of the aorta (AO). The LRA runs posterior and parallel to the left renal vein (LRV), toward the left renal hilum (LK). (*B*) Transverse color Doppler scan of the LRA from AO, posterior to the LRV.

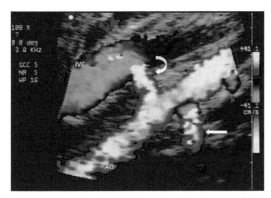

Fig. 3. Oblique coronal color Doppler image of the aorta (AO) from right anterior approach. The right renal artery *(curved arrow)* runs toward the transducer and crosses the inferior vena cava (IVC) posteriorly. The left renal artery *(straight arrow)* runs away beyond the aorta.

the segmental and interlobar arteries traverse directly toward the transducer, Doppler signal sensitivity is good, making the Doppler interrogation of intrarenal vessels relatively undemanding. A point to note at is as color Doppler signals are angle-dependant, the color of the intrarenal vessels will appear opposite in near and distal aspects of the kidney. A spectral analysis of flow is performed in the segmental branch arteries and in the interlobar arteries, systematically in upper, middle and lower parts of both the kidneys. Acceleration index (AI) and acceleration time (AT) of the systolic slope should be recorded. Care should be taken while recording the AI and AT, as often the early systolic peak does not always correspond to the peak systole. There may be a shoulder before the peak systole or an early systolic notch, and only the first slope of the systole should be measured (see **Fig. 4**).

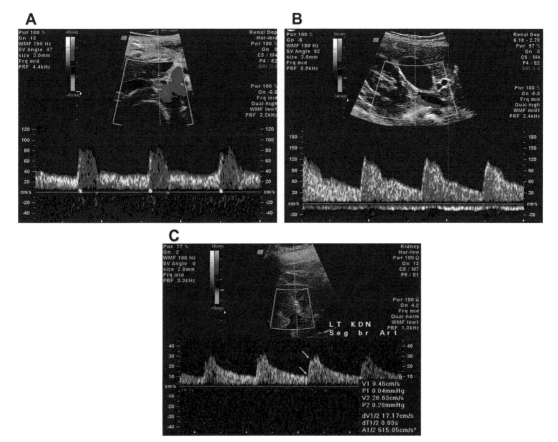

Fig. 4. Normal spectral Doppler waveforms in the renal artery. *(A)* Spectral Doppler sampling in the right renal artery origin. *(B)* Spectral Doppler sampling in mid part of the renal artery. Normal waveforms reveal a sharp systole and a good amount of diastolic flow. *(C)* Sampling in interlobar artery. Measurement of the acceleration index and acceleration time; measurements for systolic slope are recorded from the start of the slope to the top of the first peak *(arrows)*.

A renovascular Doppler study is one of the most difficult ultrasound examinations to perform, but with the present equipment, patient preparation, and meticulous technique, it is possible to achieve technically satisfactory examination in most, with a reported success rate approaching 99% as reported in a recent study using new technology.[27]

DIAGNOSIS OF RENAL ARTERY STENOSIS

Blood flow velocities increase significantly within a narrow segment, as the volume flow has to be maintained across the stenotic segment. The increase in velocity is proportional to the degree of narrowing of lumen. The aim of Doppler examination is to detect focal high velocity turbulent flow in the main renal arteries, which indicates a stenosis. This is seen as a focal region of aliasing on the color flow map. A spectral Doppler sample reveals a high PSV and broadening of the Doppler spectrum due to turbulence created at this site. A significant stenosis has a decompressing effect on the arterial flow and a dampened flow with a

tardus–parvus waveform visible beyond the stenosis. The intrarenal segmental arteries also may be targeted to detect this poststenotic phenomenon. Presently a consensus has emerged to use a double approach to diagnosis of renal artery stenosis. Direct evidence from the site of stenosis in the main renal arteries and indirect evidence from the intrarenal arteries contribute to enhancing the accuracy of Doppler examinations (**Fig. 5**).

Most observers acknowledge 1.8 to 2.0 m/s as the cut-off for PSV in the main renal artery and 3.5 as the cut-off for RAR (a ratio of the PSV in the renal artery to the PSV in the aorta) for the diagnosis of a significant renal artery stenosis. Lowering the RAR to 3.0 increases the sensitivity considerably, without affecting the specificity adversely.[28] Intrarenal parameters most commonly used are a slow upstroke of systolic acceleration, AI of less than 3.0, and an increase in AT of more than 70 milliseconds. Some observers, however, accept that eyeballing the Doppler waveform and recognizing the tardus–parvus pattern are sufficient to diagnose

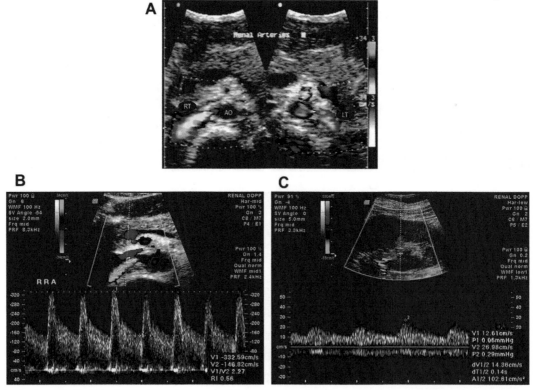

Fig. 5. Doppler findings in renal artery stenosis. (*A*) Transverse color flow image of the renal arteries as they arise from aorta (AO). Notice lumen narrowing at the origin and very bright hues of color and aliasing indicating high velocity, turbulent flow in both renal arteries. (*B*) Pulsed Doppler sampling in the narrowed artery reveals high peak systolic velocity (3.3 m/s). (*C*) Pulsed Doppler sampling in the segmental branch of a narrowed renal artery reveals a tardus–parvus waveform with abnormal parameters (AI 1.02 m/sec^2 and AT 140 ms).

poststenotic flow abnormality and that measurements of intrarenal parameters are superfluous. The calculation of the AI is influenced by the angle of insonation. Some of the studies have demonstrated that AT is the better of these two intrarenal parameters for assessing poststenotic deceleration.[29,30] There is some evidence to suggest that administration of an ACE inhibitor before a Doppler examination can improve detection of the poststenotic phenomenon, particularly the changes in the early systolic peak.[31,32]

Calculation of resistance index (RI) has been used as another indirect parameter to assess poststenotic flow in the kidneys. A side-to-side decrease in RI of more than 5% is accepted as discriminatory for significant renal artery stenosis, with a high specificity of 90% to 99%, but with low sensitivity of 30% to 77%.[25,33,34] It must be remembered that bilateral stenosis, stenosis in a single kidney, arrhythmia, and aortic regurgitation are conditions that alter the intrarenal parameters and render them unreliable for diagnosing renal artery stenosis. A renal–segmental ratio also has been proposed as a superior parameter to diagnose significant renal artery stenosis,[35] and a renal interlobar ratio has been suggested as the best parameter in diagnosing renal artery stenosis (RAS) of more than 50%.[27] These authors found a renal interlobar peak systolic velocity ratio cut-off of more than 5 and interlobar PSV of less than 15 cm/s as the best intrarenal diagnostic criteria for renal artery stenosis.[27] The contention is that in some cases the jet flow from a distal stenosis might still contaminate sampling for PSV in the segmental branch artery, but will not reach the interlobar artery, thus increasing the likelihood of recording a decreased poststenotic PSV. Using

a distal ratio instead of RAR is probably logical. With increasing degree of stenosis, the PSV in stenosis compared with the PSV in the poststenotic segment move in opposite directions. Therefore the ratio becomes much more significant, even with a slight increase in degree of narrowing (**Fig. 6**).

The use of many different criteria may be confusing to the practitioner. Most authors agree on using the double approach, of targeting the main renal arteries and the intrarenal vessels. No single parameter is good for every patient. The main renal arteries are difficult to image, but the specificity and positive predictive value of Doppler findings in the main renal artery are excellent. The flow in intrarenal vessels, on the other hand, is relatively uncomplicated to assess as compared with main renal arteries. However, it is influenced by other factors like vessel wall compliance, heart rate, and cardiac output and is not sensitive in elderly patients with known atherosclerosis (**Table 1**).

ACCESSORY RENAL ARTERY

A significant isolated stenosis of an accessory renal artery or a main renal artery branch may be associated with regional reduction in renal parenchymal thickness, identified on gray scale imaging. While examining the main arteries, imaging is performed in transverse plane superior and inferior to the main renal arteries to look for the presence of any accessory arteries. If an accessory artery is identified, flow is sampled along its length, as for the main renal artery. The sampling of intrarenal flow in all three segments of both kidneys is designed to cover the areas supplied

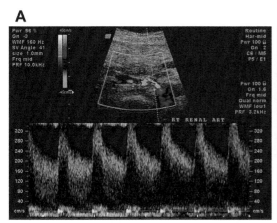
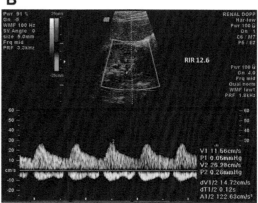

Fig. 6. Abnormal renal interlobar ratio (RIR) in renal artery stenosis. (*A*) Spectral Doppler waveform of the peak systolic velocity in the stenosis at origin of renal artery (330 cm/s). (*B*) Spectral Doppler waveform of flow in interlobar artery with a peak systolic velocity of 26 cm/s yields an abnormal RIR of 12.6.

Table 1
Doppler criteria for diagnosis of renal artery stenosis

Doppler Criteria	Main Renal Artery	Intrarenal Arteries
Direct	PSV >1.8 m/s, RAR >3.0	
Indirect		AI <3.0, AT >70 ms
Combined	RIR >5, PSV in interlobar art <15 cm/s	

Inclusion of direct evidence is preferable and diagnosis should not be based solely on indirect criteria.

Abbreviations: AI, acceleration index; AT, acceleration time; PSV, peak systolic velocity; RAR, renal aortic ratio; RIR, renal interlobar ratio.

by any accessory renal arteries. Significant difference in the waveforms among the three segments of the kidney indicates an accessory artery or branch artery stenosis (**Fig. 7**). However, there is a general apprehension that Doppler ultrasonography may miss an accessory renal artery stenosis, which is responsible for hypertension. This point has been specifically addressed by some recent studies, which concluded that an accessory renal artery stenosis is not associated with an increased risk for hypertension.[36,37] In a study of 68 stenotic renal arteries on angiography, Bude and colleagues[37] found isolated accessory renal artery stenosis in only one patient (1.5%) and concluded that failure to detect accessory renal arteries should not unduly affect the utility of a noninvasive test for detecting RVH.

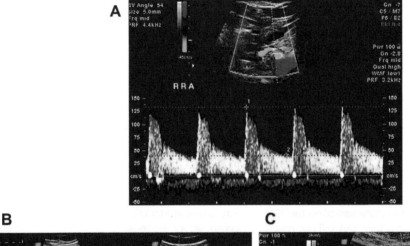

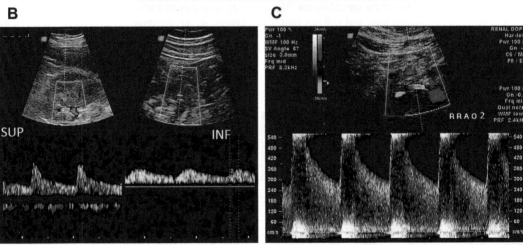

Fig. 7. Different spectral Doppler waveforms in parts of the same kidney help identify accessory renal artery stenosis. (*A*) Spectral Doppler waveform in the visualized right renal artery reveals a normal peak systolic velocity of 130 cm/s. (*B*) Spectral Doppler waveform in an intrarenal artery in upper part of kidney (SUP) reveals a normal waveform with sharp systolic peak, acceleration index (AI) 4.2 and acceleration time (AT) 20 milliseconds. Spectral Doppler waveform in an intrarenal artery of lower part of kidney (INF), demonstrates a parvus–tardus waveform, AI 1.8 and AT 170 milliseconds. (*C*) An accessory second renal artery with high velocity turbulent flow through the stenosis at the artery origin.

DISEASES UNDERLYING THE RENOVASCULAR ABNORMALITY
Atherosclerosis

Atheromatous plaques causing narrowing of the arterial lumen are the most common causes of renovascular hypertension in the elderly. The stenosis is often bilateral and most often produces a focal narrowing of the artery at its origin. The lesion develops slowly, but presentation or change in the behavior of clinical disease might be sudden. In an autopsy series, RAS ($\geq$50% stenosis) was found in 27% of patients older than 50 years; this incidence increased to 53% in those with a history of diastolic hypertension.[38] Atherosclerotic luminal narrowing may progress over time and often is associated with reduction in kidney size and function. A reduction in renal length by 1 cm per year in approximately 19% of patients with significant RAS has been observed.[39] Studies of the natural progression of disease in patients who are on medical treatment for RAS have shown that progression to arterial occlusion occurs in 9% to 16% of patients.[40,41] Atheromatous renovascular narrowing is a major cause of end-stage renal disease (**Fig. 8**).

Fibromuscular Dysplasia/Medial Fibroplasia

Arterial dysplasia is the second most common cause of renal artery stenosis and accounts for 10% to 30% of the patients with renal artery stenosis.[40] Fibromuscular dysplasia (FMD) is more common in the young and in women. FMD is described as the cause of renal artery stenosis in 30% to 60% children with RVH.[42,43] FMD produces a characteristic change in the vessel wall. Typically a string of beads appearance has been described on angiography. Usually the middle or distal segment of the artery is involved with thickening of wall. A high-velocity turbulent flow is seen on color Doppler ultrasonography. Often a color flow map might reveal irregular margins of the involved segment of the renal artery. Flow velocities are often normal in the proximal segment, which remains uninvolved (**Fig. 9**).

Aorto−Arteritis (Nonspecific Arteritis, Takayasu Arteritis)

Most Western studies record a low incidence of arteritis as a cause of renal artery stenosis, in the range of 10% to 20%,[42,44] but in developing countries, it constitutes a significant proportion. Unpublished data, 2008 from the author's own center suggests that arteritis accounts for a more than one-third of the RVH in the pediatric population. It has been reported that aorto−arteritis is the largest cause of renovascular disease in a group of children presenting with malignant hypertension.[45] Arteritis occurs most commonly in children and young adults. In the initial phase, acute inflammation may produce thickening of walls and focal dilatation of aorta, but in the late stages, fibrotic scarring produces focal stenosis, which typically involves the aorta and origins of renal arteries. Burnt out disease with residual fibrotic stenosis may be indistinguishable from aortic or renal artery ostial narrowing caused by developmental

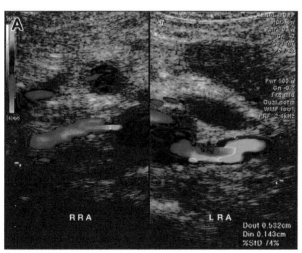
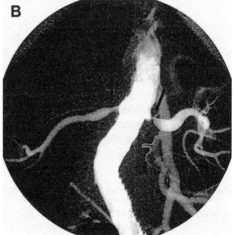

Fig. 8. Bilateral renal artery stenosis in a 57-year-old man with accelerated hypertension not controlled with three drugs. (*A*) Transverse color Doppler image demonstrates stenosis at the origins of both renal arteries. Color aliasing denotes very high-velocity flow. A poststenotic dilatation is noted in the left renal artery. (*B*) Aortogram of the same patient demonstrates the stenosis at the origin of both renal arteries (*arrows*), as well as the poststenotic dilatation in the left renal artery.

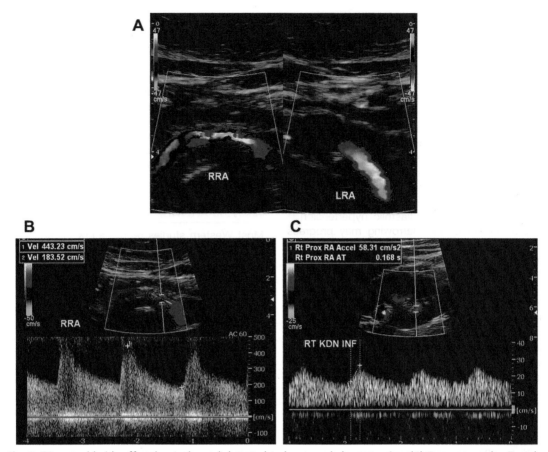

Fig. 9. 30-year-old girl suffered a stroke and detected to be severely hypertensive. (*A*) Transverse color Doppler image demonstrates narrowing of the lumen and aliasing in the middle part of right renal artery. Segmental involvement of the middle part of artery is a common feature of fibromuscular dysplasia. (*B*) Spectral Doppler waveform in the stenosis reveals a high-velocity turbulent flow with a peak systolic velocity (PSV) measured at 443 cm/s and EDV 183 cm/s. (*C*) Spectral Doppler waveform in the intrarenal artery of the affected side reveals a typical parvus–tardus waveform (acceleration index [AI] 0.58 and acceleration time [AT] 168 ms).

diseases. Arteritis very often causes bilateral RAS.[5,45] Although tuberculosis has been implicated in some cases, in a large proportion, the cause of inflammation is not apparent. Nonspecific arteritis is often a self-limiting disease, and the progression of the lesion stabilizes at some stage. Hence a simple balloon angioplasty may be useful in these cases with deployment of stents deemed superfluous (**Figs. 10** and **11**).

Neurofibromatosis and Midaortic Syndrome

Developmental renal artery stenosis is a complex disease process that affects the media with secondary intimal fibroplasia. The arterial narrowing is often indistinguishable from a stenosis caused by other diseases. Half of the patients exhibit aortic wall thickening, which causes ostial stenosis of renal arteries. In a series of 162

operations for renovascular disease, an incidence of 80% developmental disease was recorded by Stanley and colleagues (**Fig. 12**).[44] Coarctation of the aorta, William syndrome, and radiation injury to the aorta and renal arteries are other uncommon causes for renovascular hypertension.

EVALUATION FOR TREATMENT SELECTION

Surgical revascularization carries significant risks. Recently, refinement of technique and wide availability of equipment have made balloon angioplasty and placement of stents safer options. Although the technical success rates for balloon angioplasty and stent placements are excellent, quoted at 95% to 98%, not all patients benefit with complete cure of hypertension. The most common cause attributed to failure in improvement of blood pressure

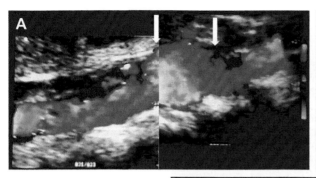
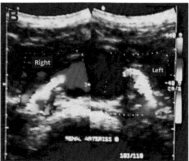
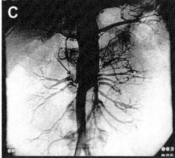

Fig. 10. 8-year-old boy, presented with pain in abdomen since 6 months. Recently has developed severe hypertension. (*A*) Mid sagittal color Doppler scan reveal a focal dilatation of abdominal aorta (*arrows*). (*B*) Transverse color Doppler scan shows ostial stenosis of both renal arteries. High velocity turbulent flow is indicated by aliasing and mosaic pattern in both renal arteries. Pulsed Doppler in Right & Left renal arteries reveals PSV of over 300 cms/sec RAR 4.0. (*C*) Aortogram confirming a fusiform segmental dilatation of aorta and ostial stenosis of both renal arteries (*arrows*), findings in early stages of aorto-arteritis.

is overestimation of the stenosis before angioplasty.[46,47] It is possible that in some patients with essential hypertension, the atheromatous plaque causing stenosis has developed later in life. Therefore the demonstration of a renal artery stenosis does not necessarily represent the cause of the patient's hypertension. An ideal test would be one with a means of assessing which patients would benefit from a revascularization procedure.

RI reflects the compliance of the vessels; therefore, it may reflect the irreversible nature of disease process. An RI of more than 0.80 predicted unfavorable outcome of revascularization in patients with RVH in one study.[24] Conversely when the RI was less than 0.80, the treatment results with angioplasty or stenting were excellent. This predictive capability has not been repeated in later studies, finding no significant difference in the outcome of patient groups with RI of more or less than 0.80.[48,49]

More recently in evaluating Doppler ultrasound and the rennin ratio, an RI cut-off of 0.80 was not found to be valuable in predicting outcome of revascularization, but it was found that severe RAS with RI of less than 0.55 responds better than moderate RAS with a high poststenotic RI.[50]

Thus it would seem rational that patients with a severe stenosis producing significant renal ischemia but without extensive glomerulosclerosis will respond better to revascularization than patients with moderate ischemia but long standing glomerulosclerosis. This would also explain why results of revascularization procedures in children and young adults are better than in those in older population.

CONTRAST-ENHANCED DOPPLER ULTRASOUND

Some data are now available about the use of ultrasound contrast in renal artery Doppler studies. The signal enhancement produced by contrast agents increases the sensitivity and specificity of Doppler ultrasonography in detection of renal artery stenosis,[51] with reports of a 25% increase in the number of RAS detected with use of contrast agents, along with a reduction in examination times.[13,52]

TRANSPLANT RENAL ARTERY STENOSIS

Stenosis of the transplant renal artery is known to cause severe hypertension and graft dysfunction.

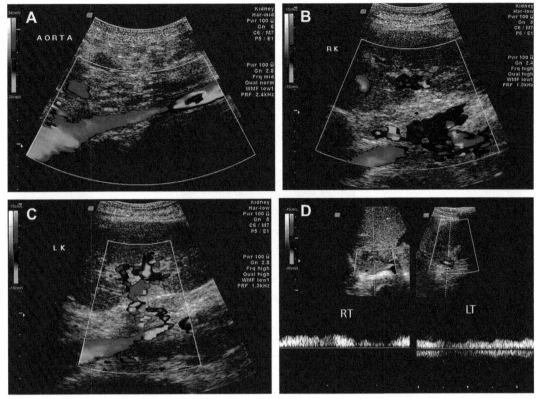

Fig. 11. 15-year-old girl with aorto–arteritis causing severe hypertension. Right kidney was 7.6 cm and left kidney 8.2 cm. There was grade 1 increase in parenchymal echogenecity. (*A*) There is thickening of the aortic walls with a significant aortic stenosis. Color Doppler image demonstrates high-velocity aliasing just beyond the stenosis. A/B ratio in aorta was 4.0 indicating a 70% to 80% stenosis. (*B, C*) Color Doppler coronal images through kidneys reveal complete obliteration of renal arteries and presence of collateral arteries supplying both kidneys. (*D*) Spectral Doppler waveform in intrarenal arteries in both kidneys revealed nonpulsatile, severely dampened flow from collaterals.

If undetected and untreated, it eventually leads to loss of the graft. Early detection and timely intervention enhance graft survival rates significantly. Stenosis develops in the transplant renal artery more commonly between 3 months to 2 years after the transplant.[53] Different timing of occurrence and location of stenosis may depend upon the underlying cause. An early stenosis developing at the anastomosis site is usually secondary to trauma to the donor or the recipient artery at the time of surgery. A late development of stenosis away from the anastomotic site may be secondary to atherosclerotic process.

As the transplanted kidney and associated artery are superficially placed structures, they are more amenable to an ultrasonographic examination. A color Doppler examination is straightforward in transplant patients, without the need of any patient preparation. Normally the iliac artery and renal artery flow are evaluated with color and spectral Doppler, with the PSV measured in the iliac artery just proximal to the anastomosis and in the renal artery just beyond the anastomosis. Accurate measurement of the PSV in the graft renal artery sometimes poses technical difficulty, particularly when there is an arterial kink. This requires operator maneuvering of the transducer placement to obtain a good angle of insonation and with it accurate Doppler angles to correctly measure velocity. This difficulty is the main cause of a range of normal PSVs reported in the transplant renal artery. The normal PSV in the proximal aspect of transplant renal artery ranges between 80 and 180 cm/s.[54] Intrarenal arteries are targeted to assess the flow patterns for poststenotic phenomena like the tardus–parvus pattern. AI, AT, and RI also are measured routinely.

The diagnosis of transplant renal artery stenosis is achieved by using similar Doppler parameters as for native renal arteries. Different criteria have

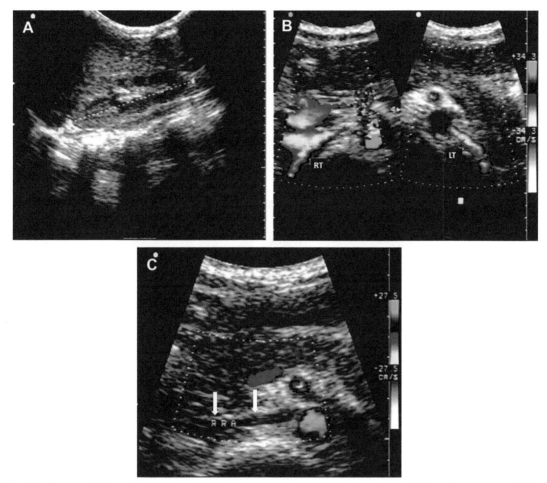

Fig. 12. 12-year-old boy with neurofibromatosis and severe hypertension. (A) Right kidney demonstrates diffuse parenchymal thinning over the lower half. (B) One right renal artery is normal in caliber and revealed normal flow. Spectral Doppler waveform in intrarenal artery in lower part of right kidney revealed parvus–tardus waveform (acceleration index [AI] 2.2 and acceleration time [AT] 97 ms). (C) Careful search, inferior to the visualized right renal artery, revealed occluded second renal artery (arrows).

been used by different workers for diagnosis of a stenosis. Baxter and colleagues[55] used a PSV of 250 cm/s; Loubeyre and colleagues[54] suggested a PSV of 180 cm/s, and recently de Morais and colleagues[56] found a transplant renal artery PSV of greater than 200 cm/s most accurate (**Fig. 13**).

INCIDENTALLY DETECTED RENAL ARTERY STENOSIS

It is not uncommon for cardiologists and radiologists to find renal artery stenosis while performing a coronary or peripheral angiography. Because atherosclerosis is a slowly progressive disease, once a lesion is documented there is a real possibility of the lesion progressing over time.[57,58] Atherosclerotic renal artery stenosis has been reported to progress at a rate of 7% per year, with the apprehension that this may eventually lead to end-stage renal disease.[57,59] In a large study, it was reported that there was a 33% incidence of significant incidental RAS in patients undergoing angiography for chronic ischemic peripheral artery disease.[60] None of these patients, however, developed end-stage renal disease on follow-up up to 10 years, questioning the suitability toward aggressive interventional treatment of incidentally detected renal artery stenosis. In a retrospective analysis of patients who had incidentally detected RAS at the time of coronary angiography, and who underwent renal artery stenting, no benefit or harm was apparent.[61] Present available evidence does not favor aggressive stenting of all the renal artery stenosis detected incidentally at the time of peripheral or

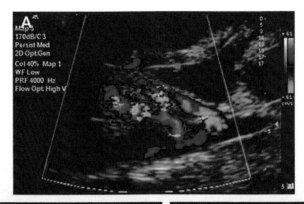

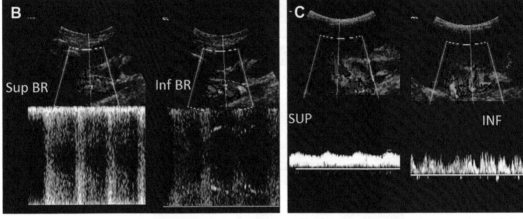

Fig. 13. 18-year-old transplant recipient developed severe hypertension 3 months following transplant. (*A*) Color Doppler scan revealed a very short main renal artery with an early bifurcation. Color aliasing and color mosaic in the two branches indicate significant stenosis at bifurcation. (*B*) Spectral Doppler waveform in the two main branches revealed very high velocity (peak systolic velocity [PSV] >280 cm/s) turbulent flow. (*C*) Spectral Doppler waveform in the segmental branches in upper and lower half of transplanted kidney revealed markedly dampened flow waveforms.

coronary angiography. A similar situation has developed with the proliferation of multidetector CT and magnetic resonance imaging (MRI) where mild or moderate renal artery stenotic lesions are detected incidentally. One must exercise a little restraint and act judiciously to assess individual cases fully before subjecting all these lesions to angiography and stenting.

MONITORING FOLLOWING REVASCULARIZATION

Doppler ultrasonography is an excellent imaging modality to monitor patients following balloon angioplasty, placement of stent, or vascular surgery. The high-velocity turbulent flow seen at the site of stenosis disappears after reconstitution of normal caliber lumen, and peak systolic velocities return to within the normal range. Similarly the tardus–parvus waveform in intrarenal arteries returns to the normal sharp systolic acceleration

after successful reopening of a stenosis. A reappearance of high-velocity, turbulent flow in the main renal artery or intrarenal tardus–parvus waveform indicates a restenosis.

SUMMARY

Color Doppler ultrasonography is an excellent screening modality for RVH. The technique is one of the most challenging ultrasound examinations; nevertheless, with expertise and skill, it is possible to perform a technically acceptable examination in most patients. The ultrasound machine technology and operator experience have constantly improved over the last decade. With evolution of the dual-access practice of targeting the intrarenal arteries along with the main renal arteries, there is a significant reduction in failed procedures and a significant improvement in overall accuracy of the technique. The advantage of Doppler ultrasonography over other imaging techniques is that it is noninvasive, inexpensive, readily available investigation that provides anatomic and physiologic information. The ideal Doppler parameters for diagnosing significant renal artery stenosis are PSV of greater than 1.8 to 2.0 m/s in the main renal artery with a renal to aortic ratio of more than 3.0. The intrarenal parameters are AI of less than 3.0 and AT of more than 70 milliseconds. A renal-to-interlobar artery PSV ratio of more than 5 and interlobar PSV of less than 15 cm/s are additional intrarenal Doppler criteria. In the future, the availability of ultrasound contrast promises to improve the sensitivity and specificity of Doppler ultrasonography in detection of renal artery stenosis. However, there is the realization that demonstration of a stenotic lesion does not always mean that it is the sole cause of patients' hypertension. In some patients, the stenosis and resultant hypertension are mild and are stable. This situation is easily controlled with medical treatment. In other patients, even use of transstenotic pressure gradient measurement and renal vein renin sampling does not guarantee a completely favorable outcome. Diagnosis and treatment options always should be exercised in view of the clinical behavior of the disease.

REFERENCES

1. Goldblatt H, Lynch J, Hanzal RF, et al. Studies on experimental hypertension of renal ischemia. J Exp Med 1934;59:347−79.
2. Conlon PJ, Athirakul K, Kovalik E, et al. Survival in renal vascular disease. J Am Soc Nephrol 1998;19: 252−6.
3. Bouyounes BT, Libertino JA. Renovascular hypertension. Curr Opin in Urol 1999;9:111−4.
4. Simon N, Franklin SS, Bleifer KH, et al. Clinical characteristics of renovascular hypertension. JAMA 1972;220:1209−18.
5. Gokhale S, Salgia P. Role of color doppler in renovascular hypertension. Ultrasound Int 2002;8: 121−6.
6. Dillon MJ. The diagnosis of renovascular disease. Pediatr Nephrol 1997;11:366−72.
7. Guzetta PC, Potter BM, Ruley EJ, et al. Renovascular hypertension in children: current concepts in valuation and treatment. J Pediatr Surg 1989;24: 1236−40.
8. Scoble JE, Hamilton G. Atherosclerotic renovascular disease: remedial cause of renal failure in the elderly. BMJ 1990;300:1670−1.
9. Svetkey LP, Himmelstein SI, Dunnick NR, et al. Prospective analysis of strategies for diagnosing renovascular hypertension. Hypertension 1989;14: 247−57.
10. Conlon PJ, O'Riordan E, Kalra PA. New insights into the epidemiologic and clinical manifestations of atherosclerotic renovascular disease. Am J Kidney Dis 2000;35:573−87.
11. Derx FH, van Jaarsveld BC, Krijnen P, et al. Renal artery stenosis towards the year 2000. J Hypertens Suppl 1996;14:S167−72.
12. Stavros T, Harshfield D. Renal Doppler, renal artery stenosis and renovascular hypertension: direct and indirect duplex sonographic abnormalities in patients with renal artery stenosis. Ultrasound Q 1994;12:217−63.
13. Lee HY, Gran EG. Sonography in Renovascular hypertension. J Ultrasound Med 2002;21:431−41.
14. Awasthi PS, Voyles WF, Greene ER. Noninvasive diagnosis of renal artery stenosis by echo Doppler velocimetry. Kidney Int 1984;25:824−9.
15. Kohler TR, Zierler RE, Martin RL, et al. Noninvasive diagnosis of renal artery stenosis by ultrasonic duplex scanning. J Vasc Surg 1986;4:450−6.
16. Taylor DC, Kettler MD, Moneta GL, et al. Duplex ultrasound scanning in the diagnosis of renal artery stenosis: a prospective evaluation. J Vasc Surg 1988;7:363−9.
17. Mirales M, Cairols M, Cotillas J, et al. Values of Doppler parameters in the diagnosis of renal artery stenosis. J Vas Surg 1996;23:428−35.
18. Puttemans T. Arterial hypertension of renovascular origin. The value of color Doppler Ultrasonography in the detection of stenosis of the renal artery. Rev Med Brux 1999;20:A341−4.
19. Handa N, Fukunaga R, Etani H. Efficacy of echodoppler examination for the evaluation of renovascular hypertension. Ultrasound Med Biol 1998;14:1−5.
20. Patriquin HB, Lafortune M, Lequier JC, et al. Stenosis of the renal artery: assessment of slowed systole in the downstream circulation with Doppler sonography. Radiology 1992;184:479−85.
21. Nazzal MM, Hoballah JJ, Miller, et al. Renal hilar Doppler analysis is of value in the management of patients with renovascular disease. Am J Surg 1997;174:164−8.
22. Desberg AL, Paushter DM, Lammert GK, et al. Renal artery stenosis: evaluation with color Doppler flow imaging. Radiology 1990;177:749−53.
23. Berland LL, Koslin DB, Routh WD, et al. Renal artery stenosis: prospective evaluation of diagnosis with color duplex US compared with angiography. Radiology 1990;174:421−3.
24. Radermacher J, Chavan A, Bleck J, et al. Use of Doppler ultrasonography to predict the outcome of therapy for renal-artery stenosis. N Engl J Med 2001;344:410−7.
25. Zeller T, Frank U, Spath M. Farbduplexsonographisch Darstellbarkeit von Nierenarterien und Erkennung hamodynamisch relevanter Nierenarterienstenosen. Ultraschall in Med 2001;22:116−21 [in German].

26. Voiculescu A, Hofer M, Hetzel GR, et al. Noninvasive investigation for renal artery stenosis: contrast enhanced magnetic resonance angiography and color Doppler sonography as compared to digital subtraction angiography. Clin Exp Hypertens 2001; 23:521–31.

27. Li JC, Wang L, Jiang YX. Evaluation of renal artery stenosis with velocity parameters of Doppler sonography. J Ultrasound Med 2006;25:735–42.

28. House MK, Dowling RJ, King P, et al. Using Doppler sonography to reveal renal artery stenosis: an evaluation of optimal imaging parameters. Am J Roentgenol 1999;173:761–5.

29. Burdick L, Airoldi F, Marana I, et al. Superiority of acceleration and acceleration time over pulsatility and resistance indices as screening tests for renal artery stenosis. J Hypertens 1996;14: 1229–35.

30. Baxter GM, Aitchison F, Sheppard D, et al. Color Doppler ultrasound in renal artery stenosis: intrarenal waveform analysis. Br J Radiol 1996;69: 810–5.

31. Oliva VL, Soulez G, Lesage D, et al. Detection of renal artery stenosis with doppler sonography before and after administration of Captopril: value of early systolic rise. Am J Roentgenol 1998;170: 169–75.

32. Quanadli SD, Soulez G, Therasse E, et al. Detection of renal artery stenosis: prospective comparison of Captopril-enhanced Doppler sonography, Captopril-enhanced scintigraphy, and MR angiography. Am J Roentgenol 2001;177:1123–9.

33. Krumme B, Blum U, Schwertfeger E, et al. Diagnosis of Renovascular disease by intra- and extrarenal Doppler scanning. Kidney Int 1996;50:1288–92.

34. Staub D, Canevascini R, Huegli RW, et al. Best duplex sonographic criteria for the assessment of renal artery stenosis—correlation with intra-arterial pressure gradient. Ultraschall in Med 2007;28:45–51.

35. de Oliveira SIRS, Widman A, Molnar LJ, et al. Color Doppler ultrasound: a new index improves the diagnosis of renal artery stenosis. Ultrasound Med Biol 2000;26:41–7.

36. Gupta A, Tello R. Accessory renal arteries are not related to hypertension risk: a review of MR angiography data. AJR 2004;182:1521–4.

37. Bude R, Forauer A, Caoili E, et al. Is it necessary to study accessory arteries when screening the renal arteries for renovascular hypertension? Radiol 2003;226:411–6.

38. Holley KE. Renal artery stenosis. A clinical pathologic study in normotensive and hypertensive patients. Am J Med 1964;37:14–22.

39. Gutzman R, Zierler R, Issacson J, et al. Renal atrophy and arterial stenosis: a prospective study with duplex ultrasound. Hypertension 1994;23:346–50.

40. Khan AN. Renal artery stenosis/renovascular hypertension eMedicine. Available at: http://emedicine. medscape.com/article/380308-overview. Accessed January, 2010.

41. Textor SC, Wilcox CS. Renal artery stenosis a common, treatable cause of renal failure? Annu Rev Med 2001;52:421–42.

42. Estepa R, Gallego N, Orte E, et al. Renovascular hypertension in children. Scand J Urol Nephrol 2001;35:388–92.

43. Broekhuizen-deGast HS, Tiel-van Bull MM, Van Beck EJ. Severe hypertension in children with renovascular disease. Clin Nucl Med 2001;26: 606–9.

44. Stanley JC, Criado E, UpChurch G, et al. Pediatric renovascular hypertension: 132 primary and 30 secondary operations in 97 children. J Vasc Surg 2006;44:1219–28.

45. Kumar P, Arora P, Kher V, et al. Malignant hypertension in children in India. Nephrol Dial Transplant 1996; 11:1261–6.

46. Leertouwer TC, Gussenhoven EJ, Bosch JL, et al. Stent placement for renal arterial stenosis: where do we stand? A meta-analysis. Radiology 2000; 216:78–85.

47. Mitchell JA, Subramanian R, White CJ, et al. Predicting blood pressure improvement in hypertensive patients after renal artery stent placement: renal fractional flow reserve. Catheter Cardiovasc Interv 2007;69:685–9.

48. Zeller T, Muller C, Frank U, et al. Stent angioplasty of severe atherosclerotic ostial renal artery stenosis in patients with diabetes mellitus and nephrosclerosis. Catheter Cardiovasc Interv 2003;58:510–5.

49. Garcia-Criado A, Gilabert R, Nicolau C, et al. Value of Doppler sonography for predicting clinical outcome after renal artery revascularization in atherosclerotic renal artery stenosis. J Ultrasound Med 2005;24:1641–7.

50. Voiculescu A, Schmitz M, Plum J, et al. Duplex ultrasound and rennin ratio predict treatment failure after revascularization for renal artery stenosis. Am J Hypertens 2006;19:756–63.

51. Drelich-Zbroja A, Jargiello T, Drelich G, et al. Renal artery stenosis: value of contrast-enhanced ultrasonography. Abdom Imaging 2004;29: 518–24.

52. Melany ML, Grant EG, Duerinckx AJ, et al. Initial experience with a phase shift ultrasound contrast agent (dodecafluoropentane) for imaging of the renal arteries. Radiology 1997;205:147–52.

53. Roberts JP, Ascher NL, Fryd D, et al. Transplant renal artery stenosis. Transplantation 1989;48:580–3.

54. Loubeyre P, Abidi H, Cahen R, et al. Transplanted renal artery: detection of stenosis with color doppler ultrasound. Radiology 1997;203:661–5.

55. Baxter GM, Ireland H, Moss JG, et al. Color Doppler ultrasound in renal transplant artery stenosis: which Doppler index? Clin Radiol 1995; 50:618–22.

56. de Morais RH, Muglia VF, Mamere AE, et al. Duplex Doppler sonography of transplant renal artery stenosis. J Clin Ultrasound 2003;31:135–41.

57. Zierler RE, Bergeline RO, Davidson RC, et al. Prospective study of disease progression in patients with atherosclerotic renal artery stenosis. Am J Hypertens 1996;9:1055–61.

58. Crowley JJ, Santos RM, Peter RH, et al. Progression of renal artery stenosis in patients undergoing cardiac catheterization. Am Heart J 1998;136: 913–8.

59. Dean RH, Tribble RW, Hansen KJ, et al. Evolution of renal insufficiency in ischemic nephropathy. Ann Surg 1991;213:446–55.

60. Leertouwer TC, Pattynama PMT, Berg-Huysmans AV. Incidental renal artery stenosis in peripheral vascular disease: a case for treatment? Kidney Int 2001;59:480–1483.

61. Zalunardo N, Rose C, Starovoytov A. Incidental atherosclerotic renal artery stenosis diagnosed at cardiac catheterization: no difference in kidney function with or without stenting. Am J Nephrol 2008;28:921–8.

Ultrasonographic Evaluation of Renal Infections

Srinivas Vourganti, MD[a], Piyush K. Agarwal, MD[a],
Donald R. Bodner, MD[a], Vikram S. Dogra, MD[b],*

KEYWORDS

- Ultrasonography • Kidney disease • Renal sonography
- Pyelonephritis

Renal sonography can be easily performed and provides valuable information concerning the underlying disease process, helping to decide appropriate management. This article reviews the important renal infections, such as pyelonephritis, emphysematous pyelonephritis, renal abscess, hydatid disease, renal tuberculosis, pyonephrosis, and human immunodeficiency virus (HIV)-associated nephropathy.

Medical ultrasonography dates back to the 1930s when it was adapted from technology used to test the strength of metal hulls of ships and applied to detect brain tumors.[1] Now with ultrasonography being performed outside of the radiology suite and in emergency departments, patient clinics, hospital rooms, and doctors' offices, it compromises approximately 25% of all imaging studies performed worldwide.[2] Ultrasonography is noninvasive, rapid, readily available, portable, and offers no exposure to contrast or radiation. Furthermore, it is easily interpretable by physicians of several different disciplines, and can result in quick diagnosis and treatment of potentially life-threatening conditions. Some of these conditions include severe kidney infections. This article focuses on ultrasonographic characteristics of various renal infections.

ULTRASONOGRAPHY PRINCIPLES

Electric waveforms are applied to piezoelectric elements in the transducer causing them to vibrate and emit sound waves. The frequency range of the sound waves emitted is above the audible human range of 20 to 20,000 Hz (cycles per second). The sound waves generated range in frequency from 1 to 15 MHz (1,000,000 cycles per second) and are directed by the transducer into the body where they are either reflected, absorbed, or refracted based on the density of the different tissues the waves pass through. Sound passes through soft tissue at an average velocity of 1540 m/s. As the sound passes through tissues of differing densities, a portion of the sound waves is reflected back to the transducer and converted into electrical signals that are then amplified to produce an image. The strength of the returning sound waves or echoes is proportional to the difference in density between the 2 tissues forming the interface through which the sound waves are traveling.[3] If the sound waves encounter a homogeneous fluid medium, such as the fluid in a renal cyst, they are transmitted through without interruption. As a result, no echoes are reflected back to the transducer, which produces an anechoic image.[4]

This article was originally published in *Ultrasound Clinics* 2006;1(1):1–13. PII: S1556-858X(05)00003-4. DOI:10.1016/j.cult.2005.09.002.

[a] Department of Urology, Case Western Reserve University School of Medicine and University Hospitals of Cleveland, 11100 Euclid Avenue, Cleveland, OH 44022, USA

[b] Department of Imaging Sciences, University of Rochester School of Medicine, 601 Elmwood Avenue, Box 648, Rochester, NY 14642, USA

* Corresponding author.

E-mail address: Vikram_Dogra@urmc.rochester.edu

ultrasound.theclinics.com

Sound waves that are strongly reflected generate strong echoes and are visualized as bright white lines, creating a hyperechoic image.

In imaging the kidney, the highest frequency that produces adequate tissue penetration with a good resolution is selected. Tissue penetration is inversely related to the frequency of the transducer. Therefore, as the frequency increases, the depth of tissue penetration decreases. Conversely, image resolution is directly related to the frequency of the transducer. Therefore, as the frequency increases, the spatial resolution of the image increases.[5] To balance these 2 competing factors, a 3.5- or 5-MHz transducer is used to image the kidneys.

ULTRASONOGRAPHY TECHNIQUE

Patients are imaged in the supine position and a coupling medium (eg, gel) is applied to the transducer to reduce the interference that may be introduced by air between the transducer and the skin. Generally a 3.5-MHz transducer is used, but a 5-MHz transducer can provide high-quality images in children or thin, adult patients. A breath-hold may be elicited by instructing patients to hold their breath at maximal inspiration. This action will displace the kidneys inferiorly by approximately 2.5 cm and may provide a better view. The right kidney can be found by placing the transducer along the right lateral subcostal margin in the anterior axillary line during an inspiratory breath-hold. If the kidney cannot be imaged because of overlying bowel gas, then the probe can be moved laterally to the midaxillary line or the posterior axillary line. Imaging the left kidney is often more challenging as it is located more superiorly, lacks an acoustic window such as the liver, and is covered by overlying gas from the stomach and small bowel. The left kidney can be localized by positioning the patient in the right lateral decubitus position and by placing the probe in the left posterior axillary line or in the left costovertebral angle.[6] The renal examination should include long-axis and transverse views of the upper poles, midportions, and lower poles. The cortex and renal pelvic regions should then be assessed. A maximum measurement of renal length should be recorded for both kidneys. Decubitus, prone, or upright positioning may provide better images of the kidney. When possible, renal echogenicity should be compared with the adjacent liver and spleen. The kidneys and perirenal regions should be assessed for abnormalities. Doppler may be used to differentiate vascular from nonvascular structures.[7]

The normal kidney appears elliptical in longitudinal view (**Fig. 1**). The right kidney varies in length from 8 to 14 cm, whereas the left kidney measures 7 to 12.5 cm. The kidneys are generally within 2 cm of each other in length and are 4 to 5 cm in width.[8] The renal cortex is homogeneous and hypoechoic to the liver or spleen. The renal sinus contains the peripelvic fat, lymphatic and renal vessels, and the collecting system, and appears as a dense, central echogenic complex. The medulla can sometimes be differentiated from the cortex by the presence of small and round hypoechoic structures adjacent to the renal sinus.[9]

RENAL INFECTIONS
Acute Pyelonephritis

A patient who has acute pyelonephritis will classically appear with localized complaints of flank pain and costovertebral angle tenderness accompanied by generalized symptoms of fever, chills, nausea, and vomiting. In addition, these findings may be accompanied by further lower urinary tract symptoms, including dysuria, increased urinary frequency, and voiding urgency.[10] Laboratory abnormalities indicative of the underlying infection can be expected, including neutrophilic leukocytosis on the complete blood count and elevated erythrocyte sedimentation rate and serum C-reactive protein levels. If the infection is severe, it may interfere with renal function and cause an elevation of serum creatinine.[11]

Evaluation of the urine will usually demonstrate frank pyuria with urinalysis, demonstrating the presence of leukocyte esterase and nitrites and microscopic findings of numerous leukocytes and bacteria.[12] However, sterile urine can be seen despite acute pyelonephritis, especially in the setting of obstruction of the infected kidney.[11] Urine cultures, which should be collected before starting antibiotic therapy, will almost exclusively demonstrate ascending infection from gram-negative bacteria. Eighty percent of infections are caused by *Escherichia coli*. The remainder of cases is mostly caused by other gram-negative organisms, including *Klebsiella, Proteus, Enterobacter, Pseudomonas, Serratia*, and *Citrobacter*. With the exception of *Enterococcus faecalis* and *Staphylococcus epidermidis*, gram-positive bacteria are rarely the cause of acute pyelonephritis.[10]

In addition to bacterial nephritis, fungal infections of the kidney are also possible. Infections with fungi are more commonly present in the setting of diabetes, immunosuppression, urinary obstruction, or indwelling urinary catheters.[12] Most commonly, *Candida* sp such as *Candida albicans* and *Candida tropicalis* are the causative organisms. In addition to the *Candida*, other fungi such as *Torulopsis glabrata, Aspergillus* sp,

A
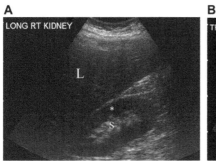

B
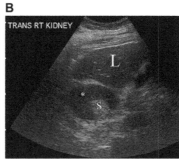

Fig. 1. Normal kidney. Longitudinal (*A*) and transverse (*B*) gray-scale sonograms of the right kidney demonstrate a hypoechoic renal cortex (*asterisk*) as compared with the liver, and a central hyperechoic renal sinus. L, liver; S, renal sinus.

Cryptococcus neoformans, Zygomycetes (ie, *Rhizopus*, *Rhizomucor*, *Mucor*, and *Absidia* spp), and *Histoplasma capsulatum* may cause renal infections with less frequency. Clinically, these infections present similarly to bacterial infections. Diagnosis can be accomplished by evaluation of the urine where fungus can be found microscopically or through fungal cultures. These infections can cause the formation of fungal balls, otherwise called bezoars, in the renal pelvis and collecting system, which can contribute to obstruction.[13]

Ultrasonographic features of acute pyelonephritis

Imaging is generally not necessary for the diagnosis and treatment of acute pyelonephritis. In uncomplicated cases, ultrasound imaging will usually find a normal-appearing kidney.[6] However, in 20% of cases, generalized renal edema attributed to inflammation and congestion is present, which can be detected by ultrasonographic evaluation. This edema is formally defined as an overall kidney length in excess of 15 cm or, alternatively, an affected kidney that is at least 1.5 cm longer than the unaffected side.[11] Dilatation of the collecting system in the absence of appreciable obstructive cause may also be detected by ultrasonography. A proposed mechanism of this dilatation is that bacterial endotoxins may inhibit normal ureteric peristaltic motion, resulting in hydroureter and hydronephrosis.[10] Parallel lucent streaks in the renal pelvis and ureter, which are most likely caused by mucosal edema, may also be detected on ultrasonography. This finding is the equivalent of a striated nephrogram appearance on computed tomography (CT). In addition, the renal parenchyma may be hypoechoic or attenuated. In cases of fungal infection, collections of air may be seen in the bladder or collecting system as the fungus may be gas-forming. In addition, ultrasonography may demonstrate evidence of fungal debris in the collecting system, such as a bezoar and consequent obstruction (**Fig. 2**).[13]

In relation to other modalities of renal imaging (Tc-99 m dimercaptosuccinic acid [DMSA] scintigraphy, spiral CT, and magnetic resonance), ultrasonography has been found to be less sensitive and specific in the diagnosis of acute pyelonephritis.[14] In the pediatric population, where a missed diagnosis can mean irreversible damage, Tc-99 m DMSA scintigraphy is still considered the gold standard of imaging.[15] Improvements in ultrasound techniques by way of power Doppler ultrasonography have resulted in better imaging than B-mode ultrasonography alone, but do not improve on the accuracy of Tc-99 m DMSA scintigraphy.[16] Some investigators suggest that although power Doppler cannot replace Tc-99 m DMSA scintigraphy because of its lack of sensitivity, a positive power Doppler ultrasonography finding can obviate the need for further imaging.[17] In addition, when combined with concomitant laboratory findings such as an elevated serum C-reactive protein level, sensitivity and specificity can be improved, and results correlate with those

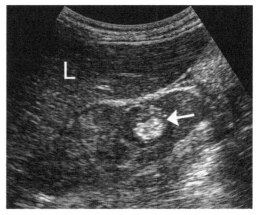

Fig. 2. Fungal ball. Longitudinal gray-scale sonogram of the right kidney in an immunocompromised patient demonstrates an echogenic mass (*arrow*) within a dilated calyx confirmed to be a fungus ball. L, liver.

of DMSA findings.[18] However, suggestions that ultrasonography can serve as a replacement for other more sensitive modalities in the detection of acute pyelonephritis remain controversial.

Acute Focal and Multifocal Pyelonephritis (Acute Lobar Nephronia)

Acute focal and multifocal pyelonephritis occur when infection is confined to a single lobe or occurs in multiple lobes, respectively, of the kidney. More common in patients who have diabetes and those who are immunosuppressed, these infections will present with clinical features similar to acute pyelonephritis. However, the patient will generally experience more severe symptoms than patients who have uncomplicated pyelonephritis. In addition, focal pyelonephritis commonly progresses to sepsis.[10] Treatment is similar to other complicated cases of acute pyelonephritis, with 7 days of parenteral antibiotics followed by a 7-day course of oral antibiotics.[11]

Ultrasonographic features of acute focal and multifocal pyelonephritis

In imaging acute focal pyelonephritis, it is important to differentiate it from the more severe case of a renal abscess that requires more aggressive management. On ultrasonography, the classic description of acute focal pyelonephritis is of a sonolucent mass that is poorly margined with occasional low-amplitude echoes that disrupt the corticomedullary junction (Fig. 3).[6] The absence of a distinct wall is a defining feature that differentiates focal nephritis from the more serious renal abscess.[19] Farmer and colleagues[20] suggest that an ultrasonographic appearance of increased echogenicity, rather than sonolucent masses, may also be commonly seen in focal nephritis. The ultrasonographic evaluation should be complemented with a CT evaluation, which is more sensitive in detecting focal pyelonephritis.[21] CT findings demonstrate a lobar distribution of inflammation that appears as a wedge-shaped area of decreased contrast enhancement on delayed images. In more severe disease, a hypodense mass lesion can be seen.[19] The radiologic appearance of multifocal disease is identical to focal disease except that it is seen in more than one lobe.

Renal Abscess

Before the advent of antibiotics, most abscesses in the kidney were caused by hematogenous spread (usually of *Staphylococcus* sp) from distant sites. These renal carbuncles would be associated with a history (often remote) of a gram-positive

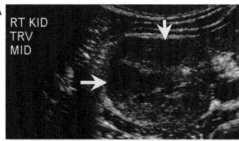

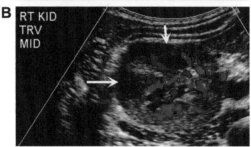

Fig. 3. Pyelonephritis. Transverse gray-scale (*A*) and color flow Doppler (*B*) sonography of the right kidney demonstrate 2 wedge-shaped areas of decreased echogenicity (*arrows*) in the renal cortex with absence of color flow, consistent with multifocal pyelonephritis.

infection elsewhere in the body, such as a carbuncle of the skin.[10] With antibiotic therapy now common, renal carbuncles are now rare, and instances of renal abscess are now primarily caused by ascending infection with enteric, aerobic, gram-negative bacilli, including *E coli*, *Klebsiella* sp, and *Proteus* sp.[19] Patients are at an increased risk for these abscesses if they have a complicated urinary tract infection (with stasis or obstruction), are diabetic, or are pregnant.[10] Patients will present with fever, chills, and pain in their back and abdomen. In addition, many will have symptoms characteristic of a urinary tract infection, such as dysuria, frequency, urgency, and suprapubic pain. Constitutional symptoms of malaise and weight loss may also be seen.[10] Laboratory studies will demonstrate leukocytosis. In nearly all renal carbuncles, and up to 30% of gram-negative abscesses, the abscess does not involve the collecting system and urine cultures will be negative.[19] In general, any positive urine culture will match the blood culture in the setting of an ascending gram-negative abscess. In the event of a gram-positive renal carbuncle, the urine culture and blood cultures may isolate different organisms from one another.[10]

The management of renal abscesses is generally dictated by their size. Small abscesses (smaller than 3 cm) are treated conservatively with observation and parenteral antibiotics.

Similar-sized lesions in patients who are immuno-compromised may be treated more aggressively with some form of abscess drainage. Lesions between 3 and 5 cm are often treated with percutaneous drainage. Any abscess larger than 5 cm usually requires surgical drainage.

Ultrasonographic features of renal abscess

Ultrasonography is particularly useful in the diagnosis of renal abscess.[19] It usually shows an enlarged kidney with distortion of the normal renal contour (**Fig. 4**). Acutely, the abscess will appear to have indistinct margins with edema in the surrounding renal parenchyma. However, after convalescence, it will appear as a fluid-filled mass with a distinct wall. This clear margin helps to distinguish this entity from the less severe focal nephritis. Once identified by ultrasonography, CT scanning with contrast enhancement can better characterize these lesions. The abscess will be seen as a round or oval parenchymal mass with decreased levels of attenuation. A ring circumscribing the lesion will form with contrast enhancement ("ring sign") because of the increased vascularity of the abscess wall.[10] In many instances, it will be difficult to definitively distinguish a renal abscess from a renal tumor. In these cases, radiologic-guided drainage with analysis of fluid can be helpful in establishing the diagnosis.

Emphysematous Pyelonephritis

Emphysematous pyelonephritis is a complication of acute pyelonephritis in which gas-forming organisms infect renal parenchyma. It is usually caused by *E coli* (70% of cases), but *Klebsiella pneumoniae* and *Proteus mirabilis* can cause emphysematous pyelonephritis with less

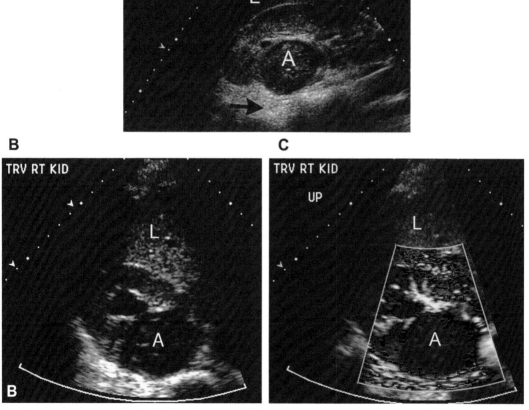

Fig. 4. Renal abscess. Longitudinal (*A*) and transverse (*B*) gray-scale sonograms of the right kidney reveal presence of a well-defined hypoechoic lesion (A) near the superior pole, with posterior through-transmission (*arrow*). Corresponding power Doppler image (*C*) demonstrates an increased peripheral vascularity. L, liver.

frequency.[22] A necrotizing infection occurs in the renal parenchyma and perirenal tissues in which tissue is used as a substrate with carbon dioxide gas released as a by-product. Clinically, this infection usually occurs in patients who have diabetes in the setting of urinary tract obstruction. Women are affected more than men. There have been no reported cases in children. Nearly all patients will present with the following triad of symptoms: fever, vomiting, and flank pain. Pneumaturia can be seen when the collecting system is involved. However, focal physical findings are commonly absent.[11]

Once discovered, prompt treatment is imperative. Management should begin with supportive care, management of diabetes, and relief of any underlying obstruction. If infection is discovered in one kidney, the contralateral kidney should also be thoroughly investigated, as bilateral involvement is seen in up to 10% of cases. The classic management for emphysematous pyelonephritis is administration of broad-spectrum antibiotics along with emergent nephrectomy.[10] Despite this aggressive therapy, mortality is seen in 30% to 40% of cases.

Ultrasonographic features of emphysematous pyelonephritis

Emphysematous pyelonephritis is diagnosed by demonstrating gas in the renal parenchyma with or without extension into the perirenal tissue.[10] Ultrasound examination will characteristically show an enlarged kidney containing high-amplitude echoes within the renal parenchyma, often with low-level posterior dirty acoustic shadowing known as reverberation artifacts (**Fig. 5**). However, the depth of parenchymal involvement may be underestimated during the ultrasound examination. Consequently, multiple renal stones may also manifest as echogenic foci without "clean" posterior shadowing,[23,24] The isolated presence of gas within the collecting system can be seen after many interventional procedures and should not be confused with emphysematous pyelonephritis. In these cases, an evaluation using CT is always warranted and is considered the ideal study to visualize the extent and amount of gas. In addition, CT can identify any local destruction to perirenal tissues. Radiologic studies play an important role in evaluation of the effectiveness of therapy in emphysematous pyelonephritis. As carbon dioxide is rapidly absorbed, any persistence of gas after 10 days of appropriate treatment is indicative of failed therapy.[10]

Pyonephrosis

Pyonephrosis is a suppurative infection in the setting of hydronephrosis, which occurs as the

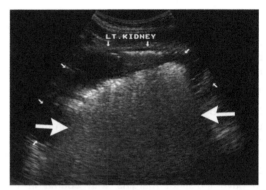

Fig. 5. Emphysematous pyelonephritis. Longitudinal gray-scale sonogram of the left kidney (*small arrows*) demonstrates air within the renal parenchyma with reverberation artifact (*large arrows*).

result of obstruction. The renal pelvis and calyces become distended with pus.[6] Patients present with fevers, chills, and flank pain. Because of the obstruction, bacteriuria can be absent. It is imperative that this obstruction is relieved through a nephrostomy or ureteral stent. If untreated, pyonephrosis can cause destruction of renal parenchyma and irreversible loss of renal function.[10]

Ultrasonographic features of pyonephrosis

Ultrasonographic findings are useful in early and accurate diagnosis of pyonephrosis. On examination, persistent echoes are seen in a dilated collecting system (**Fig. 6**). This echogenicity is caused by debris in the collecting system, and is therefore seen in dependent areas of the collecting system. Shifts in this debris can sometimes be appreciated if the patient is asked to change positions during the ultrasound examination. In addition, air can be seen in these infections. In this event, strong echoes with acoustic shadowing can be seen behind the affected area of the collecting system.[11]

Xanthogranulomatous Pyelonephritis

Xanthogranulomatous pyelonephritis (XGP) is a rare inflammatory condition that is seen in the setting of long-term and recurrent obstruction from nephrolithiasis accompanied by infection. It results in the irreversible destruction of renal parenchyma. This damage begins in the renal pelvis and calyces and eventually extends into the renal parenchyma, and can occur in either a diffuse or segmental pattern.[11] Although the cause of XGP is unknown, it is thought that the inflammatory process that occurs in response to tissue damage by bacterial infection (usually *Proteus mirabilis* or *E coli*) results in the deposition of lipid-laden histiocytes at the site of infection.

A **B**

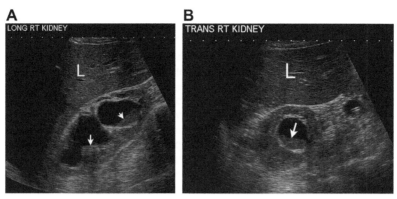

Fig. 6. Pyohydronephrosis. Longitudinal (*A*) and transverse (*B*) gray-scale sonograms of the right kidney demonstrate an enlarged hydronephrotic kidney with a fluid-fluid level (*arrows*) in the dilated calyces secondary to pus appearing as echogenic debris. L, liver.

These macrophages, or xanthoma cells, along with other inflammatory cells, result in the formation of fibrous tissue. This granulomatous process eventually replaces the adjacent normal renal parenchyma and adjacent renal tissue.[10]

Clinically, XGP is seen more commonly in women than men. Incidence peaks during the fifth to sixth decade of life. Patients who have diabetes are predisposed to the formation of XGP. Symptoms include those that suggest underlying chronic infection in the setting of obstruction, such as fever, flank pain, persistent bacteriuria, or history of recurrent infected nephrolithiasis. XGP results in the irregular enlargement of the kidney and is often misdiagnosed as a tumor. Even by pathologic examination, XGP can closely resemble malignancy, such as renal cell carcinoma. Definitive diagnosis is often made only after surgical removal, which allows thorough pathologic examination. Treatment of XGP involves surgical removal of the entire inflammatory process. Limited disease may be amenable to partial nephrectomy; however, more widespread XGP requires total nephrectomy and removal of the involved adjacent tissue.[11] Although classic management suggests that conservative intervention through simple incision and drainage commonly results in further complications, some investigators suggest this course in cases of limited focal disease.[25]

Ultrasonographic features of xanthogranulomatous pyelonephritis

Definitive preoperative diagnosis is extremely difficult to establish in XGP. By ultrasonographic evaluation, multiple hypoechoic round masses can be seen in the affected kidney. These masses can demonstrate internal echoes and can be abscesses (with increased sound through-transmission) or solid granulomatous processes (with decreased sound through-transmission).[11] Global enlargement with relative preservation of the renal contour can be seen with diffuse disease. However, in focal or segmental XGP a mass-like lesion may be appreciated. In addition, evidence of obstruction and renal calculus is commonly seen (85%).[26] In general, CT evaluation is considered more informative than ultrasonography in describing XGP. A large reniform mass within the renal pelvis tightly surrounding a central calcification is seen on CT imaging.[10] Dilated calyces and abscesses that replace normal renal parenchyma will appear as water-density masses. Calcifications and low-attenuation areas attributed to lipid-rich xanthogranulomatous tissue may be seen within the masses.[27] If contrast is used, a blush is seen in the walls of these masses because of their vascularity. This enhancement, which is limited to the mass wall only, will help distinguish XGP from renal tumors and other inflammatory processes that do enhance throughout.[11]

Renal Malakoplakia

Renal malakoplakia is a rare inflammatory disorder associated with a chronic coliform gram-negative urinary tract infection (usually *E coli*) resulting in the deposition of soft, yellow-brown plaques within the bladder and upper urinary tract. The cause is thought to be abnormal macrophage function that causes incomplete intracellular bacterial lysis. This lysis results in the deposition of histiocytes, called von Hansemann cells, which are filled with these bacteria and bacterial fragments. The bacteria form a nidus for calcium phosphate crystals, which form small basophilic bodies called Michaelis-Gutmann bodies.[10]

Clinically, malakoplakia of the urinary tract usually occurs in women. Most patients are older than 50 years. There is often an underlying condition compromising the immune system, such as diabetes, immunosuppression, or the presence of a chronic debilitating disease. Symptoms of a urinary tract infection may be present, such as fever, irritative voiding symptoms, and flank pain. In addition, a palpable mass may be appreciated.[11] If the disease involves the bladder, symptoms of bladder irritability and hematuria may be seen.

Ultrasonographic features of malakoplakia

Imaging findings of malakoplakia are nonspecific and can often mimic other pathology, such as renal tumors.[28] The most common ultrasonographic feature of renal malakoplakia is diffuse enlargement of the affected kidney.[29] Increased echogenicity of the renal parenchyma can be seen because of a confluence of the plaques.[10] In addition, hypoechoic lesions and distortion of parenchymal echoes may be appreciated.[29]

Hydatid Disease of the Kidney (Renal Echinococcosis)

Echinococcosis is a parasitic infection that is most commonly seen in South Africa, the Mediterranean, Eastern Europe, Australia, and New Zealand. It is caused by the tapeworm *Echinococcus granulosis*. Although the adult form is zoonotic, mostly found in the intestines of dogs, humans may serve as an intermediate host of this parasite while it is in the larval stage.[11] Infection more commonly manifests in the liver and lungs, with only 4% of echinococcosis involving the kidney, because the larvae, which originally invade the body through the gastrointestinal tract, must first escape sequestration in the liver and subsequently the lungs. Only after these 2 defenses are surpassed are the larvae able to gain widespread access to the systemic circulation and, correspondingly, the kidneys.[30]

The offending lesion will most commonly form as a solitary mass in the renal cortex. It is divided into 3 distinct zones. The outermost adventitial layer consists of host fibroblasts that may become calcified. A middle laminated layer consists of hyaline that surrounds a third inner germinal layer. The germinal layer is composed of nucleated epithelium and is where the echinococcal larvae reproduce. The larvae attach to the surrounding germinal layer and form brood capsules. These brood capsules grow in size and will remain connected to the germinal layer by a pedicle for nutrition. The core of this hydatid cyst contains detached brood capsules (daughter cysts), free larvae, and fluid, a combination known as hydatid sand.[10]

Clinically, most patients who have renal echinococcosis are asymptomatic, especially in the beginning stages of the disease process, because the cyst starts small and grows at a rate of only 1 cm annually. Because of their focal nature, small hydatid cysts will rarely affect renal function. As the lesion progresses, a mass effect will contribute to symptoms of dull flank pain, hematuria, and a palpable mass on examination.[10] If the cyst ruptures, a strong antigenic immune response ensues with possible urticaria and even anaphylaxis.[30] If a cyst ruptures into the collecting system, the patient will develop symptoms of hydatiduria, including renal colic and passage of urinary debris resembling grape skins.[11]

Treatment of echinococcal disease in the kidney is primarily surgical. Medical therapy with antiparasitic agents, such as mebendazole, has been shown to be largely unsuccessful. In removing a cyst, great care must be taken to avoid its rupture. Any release of cyst contents can contribute to

Table 1
Gharbi ultrasonographic classification of hyatid cysts

Type	Pathology	Frequency	Ultrasonographic Findings
I	Discrete univesicular mass	22%	Liquid-filled cyst with parietal echo backing
II	Univesicular mass with detached membranes	4%	Liquid-filled cyst with ultrasonographic water lily sign
III	Multivesicular mass	54%	Partitioned cyst with a spoke wheel appearance
IV	Heterogeneous mass	12%	Heterogeneous echo structure with mixed solid and liquid components
V	Heterogeneous mass with calcifications	8%	Dense reflections with a posterior shade cone caused by calcifications

anaphylaxis. In addition, the release of the larvae can result in the dissemination of the disease. In the event of rupture, or if resection of the entire cyst is not possible, careful aspiration of the cyst is indicated. After the contents of the cyst are removed, an infusion of an antiparasitic agent (eg, 30% sodium chloride, 0.5% silver nitrate, 2% formalin, or 1% iodine) is reinfused into the cyst.[11]

Ultrasonographic features of renal echinococcosis

Ultrasonographic findings of echinococcosis demonstrate different findings based on the age, extent, and complications of the hydatid cyst.[30] These lesions can be classified by the Gharbi ultrasonographic classification (**Table 1**).[30] The Gharbi classification assists in the characterization of renal masses that are caused by hydatid disease. Higher Gharbi type corresponds with further disease progression. Consequently, Gharbi type I cysts are most commonly seen in children. Accordingly, Gharbi types III through V are consistent with more advanced disease and are seen almost exclusively in adults. Most common are the Gharbi type III cysts, which are multivesicular masses that can be detected on ultrasonography as a partitioned cyst with a spoke wheel appearance (**Fig. 7A, B**).[31] Changes in patient position can cause any hydatid sand that is present to be disturbed and will result in the shifting of bright echoes within the mass. This finding has been described as the snowstorm sign,[11,32] Less commonly seen are the univesicular Gharbi type I and type II cysts, which demonstrate less disease progression and are seen more commonly in young adults and children. Type I cysts are well-limited liquid cysts that can be differentiated from simple nonhydatid cysts by the presence of a parietal echo. Gharbi type II cysts demonstrate a detached and floating membrane that is pathognomonic for hydatid disease. This detachment of the membranes inside the cyst has been referred to as the ultrasound water lily sign because of its resemblance to the radiographic water lily sign seen in pulmonary cysts (see **Fig. 7C**),[33,34] In contrast, the Gharbi type IV and type V cysts demonstrate more advanced disease and are correspondingly seen in older patients. Gharbi type IV hydatid cysts will demonstrate heterogeneity of echo structure with a combination of liquid and solid cyst contents. Gharbi type V hydatid cysts are calcified and will show dense reflections with a posterior shade cone. The varying echogenic aspects of these type IV and type V lesions make diagnosis by ultrasonography more difficult.[30] In these cases, CT studies can aid in characterization. On CT, the presence of smaller

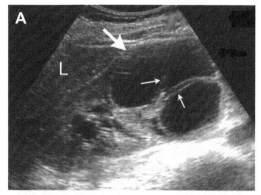

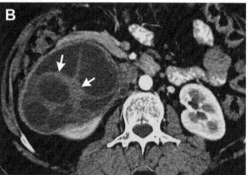

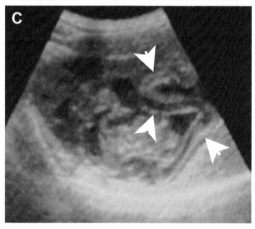

Fig. 7. Renal hydatid cyst. Gray-scale ultrasonogram (A) and contrast-enhanced CT scan (B) of the right kidney reveal a well-defined cystic lesion (*large arrow*) with multiple internal septae (*small arrows*) suggestive of a hydatid cyst with multiple daughter cysts. (*Courtesy of* SA Merchant, Mumbai, India.) (C) Gray-scale sonography of the right kidney on a different patient demonstrates the floating membranes (*arrowheads*) of the hydatid cyst following rupture of the cyst, referred to as the water lily sign. (*Courtesy of* Ercan Kocakoc, Turkey.)

round daughter cysts within the mother cysts can help differentiate hydatid lesions from other similar appearing pathology, such as simple cysts, abscesses, and necrotic neoplasm.[10]

Renal Tuberculosis

Tuberculosis is an infection caused by *Mycobacterium tuberculosis*. Typically acquired by inhalation, exposure initially results in a primary infection with a silent bacillemia. This infection will result in systemic dissemination of mycobacteria. Latent foci may result in kidney lesions many years following primary infection, though only 5% of patients who have active tuberculosis will have cavitary lesions in the urinary tract.[11]

Clinically, this infection presents in younger patients, with 75% of those affected being younger than 50 years. Renal tuberculosis should be considered in any patient who has a diagnosed history of tuberculosis. Often patients will present asymptomatically, even in cases of advanced disease. If disease involves the bladder, symptoms of urinary frequency may result. One-quarter of patients will present with findings of a unilateral poorly functioning kidney. Other suspicious findings include chronic cystitis or epididymitis that is recalcitrant to treatment; firm seminal vesicles on digital rectal examination; or a chronic fistula tract that forms at surgical sites. Diagnosis of urinary tract tuberculosis can be established through a urine culture that demonstrates growth of *M tuberculosis*.

Ultrasonographic features of renal tuberculosis

Early findings of urinary tract tuberculosis are best characterized by intravenous urography. Initially, cavities appear as small irregularities of the minor calyces. These irregular changes are classically described as "feathery" and "moth-eaten." As disease progresses, it extends from the calyces into the underlying renal parenchyma. Calcifications may be appreciated in these areas of caseating necrosis. In addition, tuberculosis involvement of the ureter can result in ureteral strictures, which cause a urographic appearance of a rigid, irregular, "pipe-stem" ureter.[11] Ultrasonographic findings in the diagnosis of renal tuberculosis have traditionally been described as limited. However, recent reports describe the role of high-resolution ultrasonography in characterizing late and chronic changes in renal tuberculosis.[35] Granulomatous mass lesions in the renal parenchyma can be seen as masses of mixed echogenicity, with or without necrotic areas of caseation and calcifications (**Fig. 8**). Mucosal thickening and stenosis of the calyces is detectable by ultrasonography. In addition, findings of mucosal thickening of the renal pelvis and ureter, ureteral stricture, and hydronephrosis are seen. Finally, bladder changes such as mucosal thickening and reduced capacity are commonly detectable.

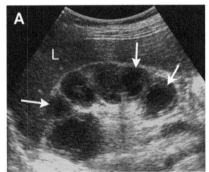
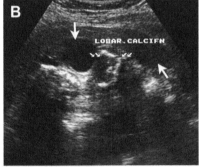
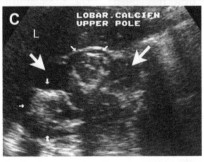

Fig. 8. Renal tuberculosis. (*A*) Longitudinal gray-scale ultrasound of the right kidney demonstrates hypoechoic areas (*arrows*) in the renal cortex suggestive of lobar caseation in this known case of tuberculosis. Longitudinal gray-scale sonography (*B* and *C*) of the kidney in another patient who has renal tuberculosis demonstrates hypoechoic areas of caseous necrosis (*large arrows*) with dense peripheral calcification (*small arrows*) with posterior acoustic shadowing. (*Courtesy of* SA Merchant, Mumbai, India.)

HIV-Associated Nephropathy

Renal disease is a common complication in patients who have HIV. This complication can result primarily from direct kidney infection with HIV or secondarily from adverse effects of the medications used to treat HIV. HIV-associated nephropathy (HIVAN) accounts for approximately 10% of new end-stage renal disease cases in the United States. Patients who have HIVAN are not typically hypertensive.

Ultrasonographic features of HIV-associated nephropathy

Sonography is a critical component in the evaluation of HIVAN. The major sonographic findings include increased cortical echogenicity, decreased corticomedullary definition, and decreased renal sinus fat (**Fig. 9**). Renal size may be enlarged.[36,37] The increased cortical echogenicity is attributable to prominent interstitial expansion by cellular infiltrate and markedly dilated tubules containing

voluminous casts. Histologically, HIVAN demonstrates tubular epithelial cell damage, glomerulosclerosis, and tubulointerstitial scarring.[38] Most patients who have HIVAN have proteinuria secondary to tubular epithelial cell damage. In the presence of marked increased cortical echogenicity in a young patient who has known history of medical renal disease, HIVAN must be considered.

SUMMARY

The growing ubiquity, well-established safety, and cost-effectiveness of ultrasound imaging have cemented its role in the diagnosis of renal infectious diseases. It is imperative that all practitioners of renal medicine understand the ultrasonographic manifestations of these diseases, as early diagnosis and treatment are the cornerstones of avoidance of long-term morbidity and mortality. If the strengths and limitations of ultrasonography are understood properly, a practitioner will be able to achieve the quickest and safest diagnosis with the minimal amount of further invasive imaging. The advent of new ultrasonographic techniques may allow it to serve a more central role in the diagnosis and characterization of renal infections.

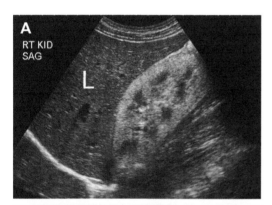

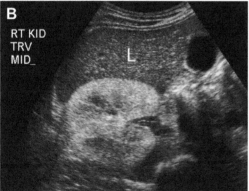

Fig. 9. HIV nephropathy. Longitudinal (*A*) and transverse (*B*) gray-scale sonograms of the right kidney in a young man who has no known history of medical disease reveals an enlarged, markedly echogenic kidney (bilateral; left not shown) with loss of corticomedullary differentiation and obliteration of sinus fat suggestive of HIV nephropathy, subsequently confirmed by histopathology. L, liver.

REFERENCES

1. Newman PG, Rozycki GS. The history of ultrasound. Surg Clin North Am 1998;78(2):179–95.
2. Harvey CJ, Pilcher JM, Eckersley RJ, et al. Advances in ultrasound. Clin Radiol 2002;57(3):157–77.
3. McAchran SE, Dogra VS, Resnick MI. Office based ultrasound for urologists. Part I: ultrasound physics, and of the kidney and bladder. AUA Update 2004; 23:226–31.
4. Spirnak JP, Resnick MI. Ultrasound. In: Gillenwater JY, Grayhack JT, Howards SS, et al, editors. Adult & pediatric urology. 4th edition. Philadelphia: Lippincott, Williams & Williams; 2002. p. 165–93.
5. Smith RS, Fry WR. Ultrasound instrumentation. Surg Clin North Am 2004;84(4):953–71.
6. Noble VE, Brown DF. Renal ultrasound. Emerg Med Clin North Am 2004;22(3):641–59.
7. Grant EG, Barr LL, Borgstede J, et al. AIUM standard for the performance of an ultrasound examination of the abdomen or retroperitoneum. American Institute of Ultrasound in Medicine. J Ultrasound Med 2002;21(10):1182–7.
8. Brandt TD, Neiman HL, Dragowski MJ, et al. Ultrasound assessment of normal renal dimensions. J Ultrasound Med 1982;1(2):49–52.
9. Horstman W, Watson L. Ultrasound of the genitourinary tract. In: Resnick MI, Older RA, editors.

Diagnosis of genitourinary disease. 2nd edition. New York: Thieme; 1997. p. 79–130.

10. Schaeffer AJ. Infections of the urinary tract. In: Walsh PC, Retik AB, Vaughn ED, et al, editors. Campbell's urology. 8th edition. Philadelphia: Elsevier; 2002. p. 516–602.

11. Schaeffer AJ. Urinary tract infections. In: Gillenwater JY, Grayhack JT, Howards SS, et al, editors. Adult & pediatric urology. 4th edition. Philadelphia: Lippincott, Williams & Williams; 2002. p. 289–351.

12. Ramakrishnan K, Scheid DC. Diagnosis and management of acute pyelonephritis in adults. Am Fam Physician 2005;71(5):933–42.

13. Wise G. Fungal and actinomycotic infections of the genitourinary system. In: Walsh PC, Retik AB, Vaughn ED, et al, editors. Campbell's urology. 8th edition. Philadelphia: Elsevier; 2002. p. 797–827.

14. Majd M, Nussbaum Blask AR, Markle BM, et al. Acute pyelonephritis: comparison of diagnosis with 99mTc-DMSA, SPECT, spiral CT, MR imaging, and power Doppler US in an experimental pig model. Radiology 2001;218(1):101–8.

15. Johansen TE. The role of imaging in urinary tract infections. World J Urol 2004;22(5):392–8.

16. Berro Y, Baratte B, Seryer D, et al. Comparison between scintigraphy, B-mode, and power Doppler sonography in acute pyelonephritis in children. J Radiol 2000;81(5):523–7.

17. Bykov S, Chervinsky L, Smolkin V, et al. Power Doppler sonography versus Tc-99m DMSA scintigraphy for diagnosing acute pyelonephritis in children: are these two methods comparable? Clin Nucl Med 2003;28(3):198–203.

18. Wang YT, Chiu NT, Chen MJ, et al. Correlation of renal ultrasonographic findings with inflammatory volume from dimercaptosuccinic acid renal scans in children with acute pyelonephritis. J Urol 2005;173(1):190–4.

19. Dembry LM, Andriole VT. Renal and perirenal abscesses. Infect Dis Clin North Am 1997;11(3):663–80.

20. Farmer KD, Gellett LR, Dubbins PA. The sonographic appearance of acute focal pyelonephritis 8 years experience. Clin Radiol 2002;57(6):483–7.

21. Cheng CH, Tsau YK, Hsu SY, et al. Effective ultrasonographic predictor for the diagnosis of acute lobar nephronia. Pediatr Infect Dis J 2004;23(1):11–4.

22. Stone SC, Mallon WK, Childs JM, et al. Emphysematous pyelonephritis: clues to rapid diagnosis in the emergency department. J Emerg Med 2005;28(3):315–9.

23. Narlawar RS, Raut AA, Nagar A, et al. Imaging features and guided drainage in emphysematous pyelonephritis: a study of 11 cases. Clin Radiol 2004;59(2):192–7.

24. Best CD, Terris MK, Tacker JR, et al. Clinical and radiological findings in patients with gas forming renal abscess treated conservatively. J Urol 1999;162(4):1273–6.

25. Bingol-Kologlu M, Ciftci AO, Senocak ME, et al. Xanthogranulomatous pyelonephritis in children: diagnostic and therapeutic aspects. Eur J Pediatr Surg 2002;12(1):42–8.

26. Tiu CM, Chou YH, Chiou HJ, et al. Sonographic features of xanthogranulomatous pyelonephritis. J Clin Ultrasound 2001;29(5):279–85.

27. Kim JC. US and CT findings of xanthogranulomatous pyelonephritis. Clin Imaging 2001;25(2):118–21.

28. Evans NL, French J, Rose MB. Renal malacoplakia: an important consideration in the differential diagnosis of renal masses in the presence of *Escherichia coli* infection. Br J Radiol 1998;71(850):1083–5.

29. Venkatesh SK, Mehrotra N, Gujral RB. Sonographic findings in renal parenchymal malacoplakia. J Clin Ultrasound 2000;28(7):353–7.

30. Zmerli S, Ayed M, Horchani A, et al. Hydatid cyst of the kidney: diagnosis and treatment. World J Surg 2001;25(1):68–74.

31. von Sinner WN. New diagnostic signs in hydatid disease; radiography, ultrasound, CT and MRI correlated to pathology. Eur J Radiol 1991;12(2):150–9.

32. Marti-Bonmati L, Menor Serrano F. Complications of hepatic hydatid cysts: ultrasound, computed tomography, and magnetic resonance diagnosis. Gastrointest Radiol 1990;15(2):119–25.

33. Beggs I. The radiology of hydatid disease. AJR Am J Roentgenol 1985;145(3):639–48.

34. Moguillanski SJ, Gimenez CR, Villavicencio RL. Radiología de la hidatidosis abdominal. In: Stoopen ME, Kimura K, Ros PR, editors. Radiología e imagen diagnóstica y terapéutica: abdomen, vol. 2. Philadelphia: Lippincott, Williams & Wilkins; 1999. p. 47–72.

35. Vijayaraghavan SB, Kandasamy SV, Arul M, et al. Spectrum of high-resolution sonographic features of urinary tuberculosis. J Ultrasound Med 2004;23(5):585–94.

36. Di Fiori JL, Rodrigue D, Kaptein EM, et al. Diagnostic sonography of HIV-associated nephropathy: new observations and clinical correlation. AJR Am J Roentgenol 1998;171(3):713–6.

37. Atta MG, Longenecker JC, Fine DM, et al. Sonography as a predictor of human immunodeficiency virus-associated nephropathy. J Ultrasound Med 2004;23(5):603–10.

38. Hamper UM, Goldblum LE, Hutchins GM, et al. Renal involvement in AIDS: sonographic-pathologic correlation. AJR Am J Roentgenol 1988;150(6):1321–5.

Ultrasonography of Genitourinary Tuberculosis

S. Boopathy Vijayaraghavan, MD, DMRD

KEYWORDS

- Sonography • Genitourinary • Tuberculous • High resolution
- Parenchymal granuloma • Parenchymal cavity

Genitourinary tuberculosis is the second most common form of extrapulmonary tuberculosis after lymph node involvement[1–3] and may account for between 30% and 41% of nonpulmonary cases. Genitourinary tuberculosis is a disease among young adults, with 60% of the affected patients between the ages of 20 and 40 years,[4] with a slight male predominance.[5] Renal involvement is rare before the age of 20 years, and signs and symptoms are usually found before the age of 40 years.[6] The kidney is usually the primary organ infected in urinary disease, and other parts of the urinary tract become involved by direct extension. The epididymis in men and the fallopian tubes in women are the primary sites of genital infection.[7] After the kidney, the next most frequently involved organs are the urinary bladder, fallopian tubes, and scrotum.[8] With the human immunodeficiency virus epidemic, an increasing number of extrapulmonary tuberculosis cases have been reported.[9,10]

URINARY TRACT TUBERCULOSIS
Pathology

Renal tuberculosis infection progresses in 2 phases, with an initial seeding of the bacteria and a subsequent delayed reactivation. At the time of initial pulmonary infection, diffuse hematogenous dissemination occurs in approximately 25% of the cases.[2,11] The bacilli become trapped in the periglomerular capillaries and form numerous small abscesses in both kidneys (at this early stage, the cortical lesions are too small to be imaged).[12,13] If the cellular immunity of the host is intact or if antituberculous chemotherapy has been administered for clinically active primary tuberculosis, the organisms remain confined to the cortex with the subsequent formation of multiple small healed granulomas. However, if host immunity is impaired, reactivation may occur between 5 and 25 years after the initial pulmonary infection.[2]

The primary cortical foci, on reactivation, spill organisms into the renal tubules and these organisms propagate to the papillae through the loop of Henle.[14] In the renal medulla, bacillary proliferation leads to the formation of granulomas, which on progression produce coalescent granulomas. The coalescent granulomas can caseate and result in parenchymal cavities, which can rupture into a calyx. Rarely, the parenchymal cavity can extend and rupture outward producing a perinephric abscess, which can later form a fistula to the skin. When the cavity ruptures into a calyx,[2] the disease can spread distally by seeding through the urothelial submucosa and lymphatic vessels to the infundibula, renal pelvis, ureter, and urinary bladder. The uroepithelium becomes inflamed, edematous, and ulcerated containing multiple tiny granulomata in its mucosa and submucosa. The most severely affected are the sites of anatomic narrowing, namely, the infundibula of the calyces, the pelviureteric junction, and the vesicoureteric junction.[2,11,15] In the urinary bladder, the initial changes consist of cystitis with

Some Text: Adapted from the article by the authors; Vijayaraghavan SB, Kandasamy SV, Arul M, et al. Spectrum of high-resolution sonographic features of urinary tuberculosis. J Ultrasound Med 2004;23(5):585–94; with the permission of the American Institute of Ultrasound Medicine.

Sonoscan: Ultrasonic Scan Centre, 15 B Venkatachalam Road, R.S. Puram, Coimbatore 641 002, Tamil Nadu, India

E-mail address: sonoscan@vsnl.com

Ultrasound Clin 5 (2010) 367–378
doi:10.1016/j.cult.2010.07.001

ulceration, inflammation, and edema of the mucosa. With generalized involvement, the capacity of the bladder is reduced.

Urinary tuberculosis is characterized histopathologically by 2 basic processes including destruction and then subsequent healing by fibrosis, with granuloma formation and calcification.[2,15]

Clinical Features

Patients with tuberculosis of the upper urinary tract are usually asymptomatic. Some may have recurrent or resistant urinary tract infections or a sterile pyuria with or without hematuria[16] (the hematuria can be macro- or microscopic).[17] Some patients may present with flank pain caused by hydronephrosis secondary to obstruction or a perinephric abscess. One uncommon manifestation is that of a flank sinus caused by a nephrocutaneous fistula, and very rarely a patient may present with renal failure when there is bilateral renal or ureteric involvement. When the urinary bladder is involved, patients commonly complain of dysuria, frequency, nocturia, suprapubic pain, and hematuria. The symptoms are chronic and intermittent, running for months and even years in some patients.

Ultrasonographic Features

The various lesions of urinary tuberculosis are well demonstrated on ultrasonography, particularly with high-frequency high-resolution ultrasound using a transducer imaging at 5 to 12 MHz, using recently introduced techniques such as compound and harmonic imaging. The ultrasonographic features of urinary tuberculosis accurately reflect the pathologic processes. An important feature of urinary tuberculosis is the demonstration of involvement of multiple areas of the urinary tract in different stages of the disease in the same patient.

The coalescent granulomas in the renal parenchyma are seen as masses of variable size and echogenicity[5,18–20] (usually mixed echogenicity), with or without necrotic areas of caseation, cavitation, and evidence of calcification (**Fig. 1**).[21] Some of these coalescent granulomas can lie very close to the calyces causing distortion. When the cavity ruptures into a calyx, the communication is seen as an anechoic tract between the parenchymal cavity and the calyx (**Fig. 2**).[18,21] When there is marked destruction of the papilla, the resulting cavity can be seen to have a broad communication in continuity with the calyx. Rarely, the sloughed necrosed papilla can even be seen in the cavity. Very occasionally the cavity can extend externally and rupture into the perinephric space, which is seen as a perinephric abscess on ultrasonography (**Fig. 3**A). The cavity may extend further into the abdominal wall (see **Fig. 3**B), eventually rupturing externally resulting in a nephrocutaneous fistula, characterized by a hypoechoic tract (see **Fig. 3**C) running from the perinephric space to the skin.[2,21]

The involvement of the collecting system is seen as varying degrees of irregular mucosal thickening in the calyces and pelvis (**Fig. 4**). It is secondary to inflammation, granuloma formation, caseation, and ulceration of the urothelium. The lesions are seen at the sites of anatomic narrowing as previously described.[2,11,15,21] In the ureter, the lesions are seen as areas of mucosal thickening with narrowing of the lumen and proximal dilatation (**Fig. 5**). If multiple sites of the ureter are involved, the lumen of the ureter has a beaded appearance caused by alternate areas of mucosal thickening (**Fig. 6**) and dilatation.[21]

A characteristic of tuberculosis is that along with these destructive features, the consequences of healing by fibrosis and calcification are seen simultaneously.[2,15] Parenchymal scars can form with or without calcification, and the healing of

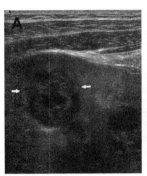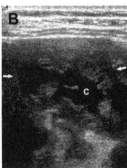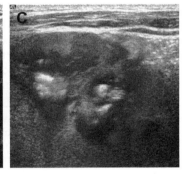

Fig. 1. (*A*) A renal parenchymal mass (*arrows*) of mixed reflectivity in keeping with tuberculosis. (*B*) A large irregular parenchymal cavity (*C*) within an echo-poor mass (*arrows*). (*C*) Kidney showing parenchymal masses containing calcification.

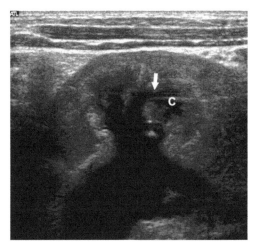

Fig. 2. Kidney showing an irregular medullary cavity (C) communicating with the calyx via an anechoic tract (*arrow*).

a parenchymal cavity may result in a tiny parenchymal cyst containing milk of calcium. The fibrous scarring of the collecting system when involving the infundibulum of the calyx produces focal caliectasis, whereas if there is a stricture of the pelvis, the characteristic feature is that of uneven or asymmetric caliectasis, in which some calyces are grossly dilated, some slightly dilated, and some not dilated at all. If all the calyces are involved, asymmetric or symmetric dilatation of all the calyces without dilatation of the renal pelvis (**Fig. 7**) can be seen. The fibrosis of the involved parenchyma, infundibulum, and renal pelvis results in variable degrees of retraction and dilatation of the kidney with kinking and distortion of the renal pelvis, the so-called Kerr kink (**Fig. 8**).[21–23] Fibrotic healing of the pelviureteric junction can result in hydronephrosis or pyonephrosis, whereas in the ureter, fibrosis can lead to single or multiple strictures with hydronephrosis. In the lower ureter, fibrotic healing can eventually result in a ureter that appears as a straight rigid tube with a patulous ureteric orifice and vesicoureteric reflux (**Fig. 9**).[14,22]

In the urinary bladder, tubercles that are formed in the mucosa can coalesce and produce ulceration and edema, with the common sites of involvement being around the ureteric orifices, where edema in the trigonal mucosa causes ureteric obstruction (**Fig 10**). Extensive involvement of the bladder mucosa results in a potentially reversible decrease in the capacity of the urinary bladder, most probably a result of spasm. The inflammation can then progress to involve the muscular layer with mural fibrosis, causing the bladder to become markedly thickened and contracted resulting in the

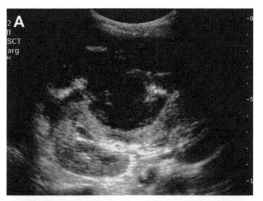

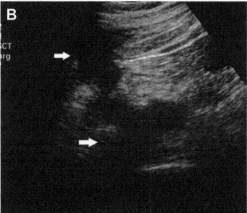

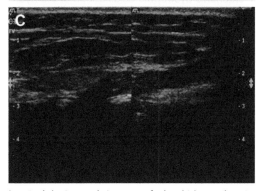

Fig. 3. (*A*) Coronal image of the kidney showing a renal and perinephric abscess. (*B*) Left flank showing extension of a tuberculous perinephric abscess into the posterior abdominal wall (*arrows*). (*C*) Left flank shows an echo-poor tract extending to the perinephric space from the skin.

so-called thimble bladder, which is not reversible (**Fig. 11**). Fibrosis in the region of the trigone may also produce gaping of a ureteric orifice and vesicoureteric reflux.[14,22] Calcification of the lesions, a part of the healing process, is seen in the renal parenchyma as clumps of punctate calcification or a lobar type of calcification deep to a scar. When the dystrophic calcifications are diffuse

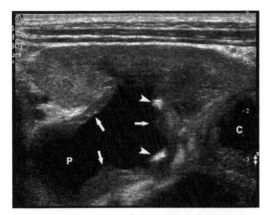

Fig. 4. Transverse view of the kidney demonstrating mucosal thickening (*arrows*) of the calyces and pelvis (P). There is calcification of the wall of a calyx and the pelvis (*arrowheads*). A parenchymal cavity (C) is also seen.

and uniform, they are described as being puttylike, a characteristic feature of renal tuberculosis, and when the calcification becomes extensive, the appearance is called putty kidney (**Fig. 12**). In the collecting system, when focal, the calcification is seen as speckled or curvilinear in the wall of the calyx, pelvis, and ureter (see **Fig. 4**). There can be extensive dystrophic calcification of the hydronephrotic nonfunctioning kidney, resulting in a cast of the kidney being formed, which is referred to as an autonephrectomy (**Fig. 13**).[2,11,24]

The confirmation of the diagnosis of urinary tract tuberculosis is made by seeing the bacilli in a smear of urine, by growth of bacilli in a urine culture, or by biopsy of lesions in the urinary bladder. If there is obstruction, for example,

ureteric stricture, the sample of urine obtained for analysis should be collected proximal to the obstruction.

Although ultrasonography can visualize a myriad of conditions caused by urinary tuberculosis, each of these can be caused by other disease processes such as other forms of papillary necrosis, malignant lesions of the kidney and collecting system, and bacterial cystitis. The major distinguishing feature of urinary tuberculosis on ultrasonography is the involvement of multiple areas of the urinary tract, with visualization of different stages of the disease in the same patient alongside a chronic course for the disease symptoms.[21]

GENITAL TRACT TUBERCULOSIS

The primary site for infection of the genital tract is often the epididymis in men and the fallopian tubes in women. Spread is via the hematogenous route with the infection spreading to adjacent organs by direct extension.[25] The sexual transmission of genital tuberculosis is very rare despite that men with genital tuberculosis can have the organisms in their semen.[26]

Male Genital Tract

Prostate
The prostate gland is the next most commonly affected organ in men, usually spreading hematogenously, with direct extension of the disease from urinary tuberculosis not having been established.[27] The disease is characterized pathologically by areas of focal necrosis with caseation

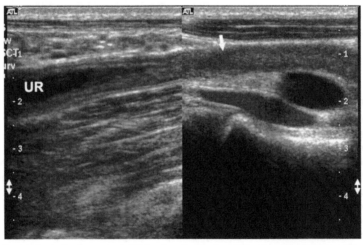

Fig. 5. Midureter showing marked mucosal thickening (*arrow*) obliterating the lumen with a dilated proximal ureter (UR).

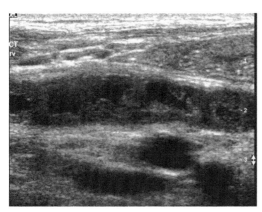

Fig. 6. Midureter showing a beaded appearance due to multiple segments of marked mucosal thickening.

and cavitation, with the lesions healing by fibrosis and calcification.[28] The fibrosis around the ejaculatory ducts can result in obstruction, leading to dilation of the proximal ductal system including the vas deferens and seminal vesicles.[29] Rarely, particularly in immunocompromised patients, there may be tuberculous abscesses of the prostate, which can extend to the periprostatic region or develop into fistulae.[30] Most patients with tuberculosis of the prostate are asymptomatic, and while some may develop hemospermia, many present with infertility, mostly with azoospermia. A rare manifestation is that of fever secondary to an abscess.

Ultrasonography of the prostate performed via the transrectal route often fails to reveal any abnormality. Occasionally, focal areas of decreased echogenicity[31,32] can be seen, as can areas of dystrophic calcification. Rarely, there may be an abscess in the prostate with or without a periprostatic collection (**Fig. 14**), which can mimic a pyogenic abscess, particularly in an

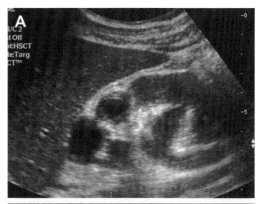

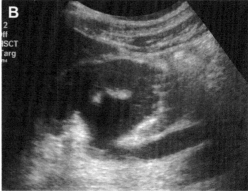

Fig. 8. (*A*) Coronal image of the kidney showing multiple parenchymal cavities in the upper pole. (*B*) On healing with fibrosis, this has resulted in distortion and kinking of the renal pelvis.

immunocompromised patient.[33] Rarely, there may be a fistulous tract to the perineum or an air-filled tract extending from the prostate to the anal canal indicating an anourethral fistula (**Fig. 15**).

When patients present with infertility due to obstruction of the ejaculatory ducts, ultrasonography shows dilated seminal vesicles associated

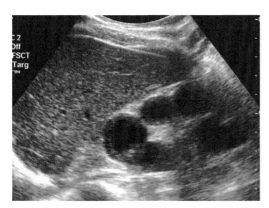

Fig. 7. Coronal image of the kidney showing dilatation of all the calyces without renal pelvis dilatation caused by a stricture of the renal pelvis itself.

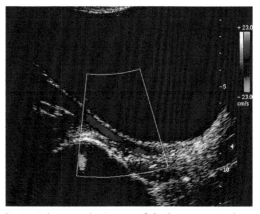

Fig. 9. Color Doppler image of the lower ureter shows vesicoureteric reflux due to healing and fibrosis.

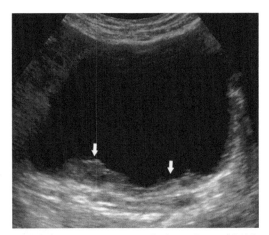

Fig. 10. Transverse image of the urinary bladder shows focal irregular mucosal thickening in the region of the trigone (*arrows*).

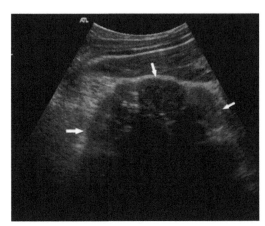

Fig. 12. Coronal image of the kidney showing the extensive calcification (*arrows*) with shadowing, characteristic of a putty kidney.

with dilated tubules in the epididymis. There may be ectasia of the rete testis and epididymal cysts. The development of prostatic lesions can be nonspecific and may mimic the appearances of malignancy or other infections. When the symptoms are chronic or there are additional features of urinary tuberculosis, a biopsy may not be necessary. Otherwise, a guided biopsy or aspiration is necessary to confirm tuberculosis. In chronic lesions that develop fibrosis and calcification, it may be impossible to prove the existence of the infection; proving the existence of infection may not even be necessary, because the treatment is directed more toward alleviating the patient's symptoms by relieving any obstruction or correcting a fistula and less so dealing with the underlying tuberculosis.[29]

Epididymal and testicular tuberculosis

Tuberculosis of the epididymis results from retrograde extension of infection from the prostate and the seminal vesicles or from hematogenous spread. Less frequently, it may be transmitted sexually or due to intravesical bacille Calmette-Guérin therapy for superficial bladder cancer.[10,33–39] Classically, the infection is said to affect the tail of the epididymis first, either because the tail has greater blood supply or because it is the first portion to be involved when there is reflux along the vas deferens.[37,40,41] However, recently Chung and colleagues[35] have suggested that the infection may in fact more frequently involve the entire epididymis or its head.

The testis may become involved secondarily by direct extension, but hematogenous spread to the

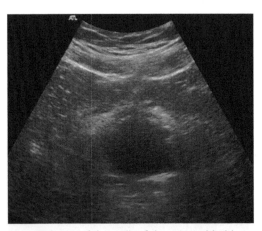

Fig. 11. Fibrosis of the walls of the urinary bladder resulting in an irreversibly thick-walled small-volume urinary bladder: thimble bladder.

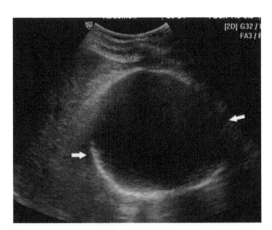

Fig. 13. Coronal image of the kidney demonstrating the calcified walls of a hydronephrotic kidney (*arrows*): autonephrectomy.

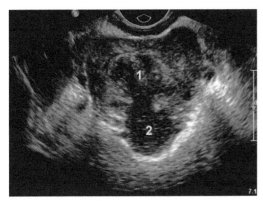

Fig. 14. Axial image of the prostate showing an abscess (1) with an extension outside the gland (2).

testis is rarely possible.[4,36,40,42,43] About 70% of patients with tuberculous epididymitis have a history of tuberculosis,[34,44,45] and although earlier reports suggested a greater incidence of bilateral involvement, recent reports have documented a higher proportion of unilateral disease.[35,37,41,46] The most common symptoms of scrotal tuberculosis are pain and swelling. Some cases are insidious and chronic, with painless or only slightly painful epididymal swelling,[10,36,42,47] but rarely, there may be a more acute presentation.[10,48,49] Although constitutional symptoms are rare,[10,46] they may occur in the presence of an abscess or sinus formation, which also indicate advanced and more widespread disease.[50] Pathologically, there is necrosis of the tubules followed by caseation and fibrosis. There are lesions in various stages of development, including exudative, granulomatous, and those healing with fibrosis,[35,46,51] with calcification

occurring later. When the tunica vaginalis is invaded, a hydrocele may develop.

Ultrasonography of the scrotum shows marked heterogeneity and correlates well with the pathologic changes such as caseous necrosis, fibrosis, granuloma formation, and calcification.[35] Tuberculous epididymitis appears as a diffusely enlarged heterogeneously hypoechoic epididymis (**Fig. 16**) or more focally with nodular heterogeneous hypoechoic lesions in epididymis (**Fig. 17**). Rarely, the epididymis is diffusely enlarged and homogeneously hypoechoic.[2,4,35,42,52] In an aggressive infection, an abscess may mimic a pyogenic infection and the abscess may extend into the scrotal wall (**Fig. 18**). When a scrotal sinus forms, an echo-poor or fluid-filled tract may extend from the epididymis (usually the tail) into the scrotal wall reaching up toward the skin surface.[35,50] The scrotal skin may become thickened, a hydrocele may form, or the patient may develop calcification of the epididymis (see **Fig. 17**) and tunica vaginalis.[35,41,42] Color Doppler ultrasonography demonstrates a few vessels in the periphery of the epididymis with absence of flow in the focal lesions.[52,53] In tuberculous orchitis, a common appearance is of an enlarged testis with multiple, small, hypoechoic nodules[35,40] or rarely there is diffuse enlargement of the testis with a homogeneous or heterogeneous hypoechoic texture[4,41,54] and occasionally, a blurred separation between the testis and epididymis (**Fig. 19**).

The differential diagnosis for scrotal tuberculosis includes acute nonspecific infection and tumors.[42,54–56] The presence of both epididymal and testicular lesions is suggestive of an infection. In cases of nonspecific infection, the clinical picture is of an acute process and the involvement is diffuse and homogeneous as opposed to tuberculosis, which characteristically has a more chronic nature with focal heterogeneous lesions.

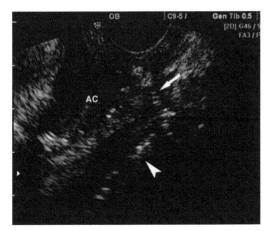

Fig. 15. Sagittal image at the level of the anal canal (AC) shows a gas-filled fistulous tract (*arrow*) between the urethra (*arrowhead*) and the anal canal.

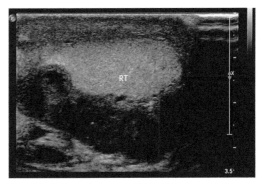

Fig. 16. Tuberculous epididymitis appearing as a diffusely enlarged, heterogeneously hypoechoic epididymis. RT, right testis.

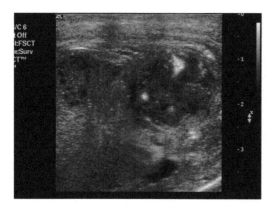

Fig. 17. Image showing a focal nodular heterogeneous lesion in the tail of the epididymis with calcification.

Occasionally, the differentiation may be difficult, but the presence of a sinus tract, the lack of response to antimicrobial agents, and any evidence of tuberculosis in the rest of the genitourinary system might help differentiate the conditions.[35] When a solitary lesion is found in the testis, it has to be differentiated from a tumor by histologic analysis.[57]

Tuberculosis of seminal vesicles and vasa deferentia

The tuberculous involvement of the seminal vesicles is the rarest form of extrapulmonary tuberculosis.[58] It occurs by hematogenous spread or secondary involvement from prostatic infection. The course is insidious and patients are usually asymptomatic with eventual development of fibrosis and calcification. The disease is usually bilateral and spreads contiguously to involve the vasa deferentia, in which case, the patient may present initially with a low-volume ejaculate and later with infertility and a finding of aspermia. A

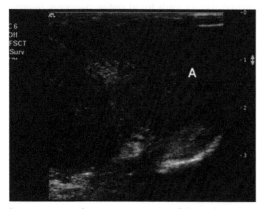

Fig. 18. Image showing extension of the tuberculous lesion of the tail of the epididymis into the scrotal wall with an abscess in the wall (A).

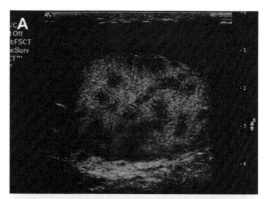

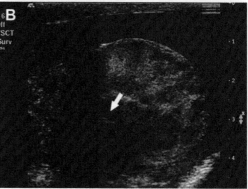

Fig. 19. (A) Image showing an enlarged testis with multiple small hypoechoic nodules and a surrounding hydrocele. (B) Diffusely enlarged testis with a heterogeneous hypoechoic texture and a blurred interface between the testis and the epididymis (arrow).

transrectal ultrasonography (TRUS) reveals small solid seminal vesicles with or without calcifications. There may be single or multiple hypoechoic masses in the vas deferens within the spermatic cord and possible calcification of the vas deferens (Fig. 20). Fibrotic atrophic seminal vesicles with aspermia have been considered a diagnostic feature of tuberculosis, and patients with such a finding need not be further evaluated and are treated with assisted reproduction.[59] The only other condition to be considered in differential diagnosis is that of congenital absence of the vas deferens, which shows an absent seminal vesicle and vas deferens on TRUS.[60] Rarely, when there is severe infection, particularly in immunocompromised patients, an abscess of the seminal vesicle may be seen, which usually also involves the prostate (see Fig. 20). These immunocompromised patients may present with fever and irritative voiding symptoms, and in such patients, TRUS is diagnostic of an abscess that is seen as an enlarged seminal vesicle with fluid and debris-filled areas within. There may be involvement of the prostate and loss of the interface between the seminal

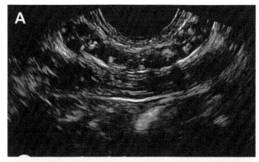

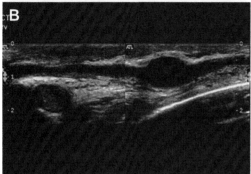

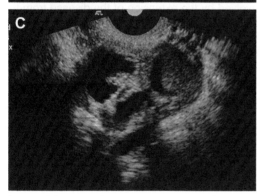

Fig. 20. (A) Image showing extensive calcification in both the seminal vesicles. (B) Image showing a hypoechoic mass associated with a vas deferens in the spermatic cord as a result of tuberculosis. (C) Seminal vesicle and prostate showing an irregular solid and cystic mass suggestive of an abscess in the seminal vesicle, which involves the prostate and indents the urinary bladder.

vesicle and the prostate and possibly thickening of the adjacent wall of the urinary bladder.[61] The findings mimic a pyogenic abscess, and an ultrasound-guided aspiration gives proof of the underlying diagnosis of tuberculosis.

Female Genital Tract

The fallopian tube is the primary site of infection in the female genital tract and the usual route is again hematogenous. Occasionally, lymphatic spread from peritoneal seeding or direct extension from

an intestinal lesion can occur.[62] The fallopian tubes are affected in 94% of women with genital tuberculosis, and in most patients, there is bilateral but asymmetrical tubal involvement. The fallopian tubes are thickened with caseous ulceration of the mucosa, resulting in ragged contours and diverticular outpouching of both the isthmus and ampulla.[63] As the tube heals, it becomes encased in connective scar tissue, and the lumen develops a beaded appearance due to multiple strictures or a rigid pipestem contour.[64] Obstruction of the fallopian tube may result in hydrosalpinx,[65] and in the late stages of disease, there may be calcification of the tubes in the form of linear streaks or tiny nodules. Tubal tuberculosis spreads to the endometrium in about 50% of cases.[64]

Pathologically, there are 2 types of pelvic tuberculosis in women: wet and dry (adhesive).[66–68] In the wet type, there is ascites and the peritoneum of the parietal wall and viscera is covered with innumerable small tubercles. The fallopian tubes, in addition to being covered with miliary tubercles on the serosal surface, are usually slightly enlarged and distended. In contrast to other forms of salpingitis, the fimbriae may be patent. Within the tubal wall and mucosa, the histologic findings are typical of tuberculosis, with tubercle formation, multinucleated giant cells, and an epithelioid reaction. In advanced cases, frank caseation is present. Dry (adhesive) tuberculosis may represent the healed fibrotic consequence of the wet ascitic pattern. The pelvic organs show evidence of tuberculous salpingitis with enlargement of the tubes and occasionally pyosalpingitis and even tuboovarian abscess formation. The clinical presentations of pelvic tuberculosis in women are extremely varied. They may present with ascites, pelvic pain, or a pelvic mass with or without constitutional symptoms. Some patients may present with infertility.

Ultrasonography demonstrates ascites, when present, which is usually septated,[68] with the septation appearing latticelike (**Fig. 21**). There may be echogenic particles in the ascitic fluid and thickening of the greater omentum and parietal and visceral peritoneum. The fallopian tubes may be thickened and seen to be floating in the ascitic fluid (see **Fig. 21**). With adhesions, the ascites may be loculated with thick septa, mimicking an ovarian tumor or tubo-ovarian abscess. In the dry type, the fallopian tubes may show thick walls (**Fig. 22**) and a distended lumen, with preserved patency on saline infusion sonohysterography. There may be a hydrosalpinx on both sides, as the involvement of the fallopian tubes is usually bilateral. Most of these features are seen in ovarian carcinoma or other infections. The occurrence of

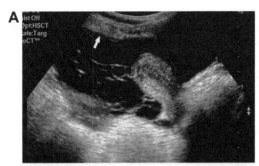

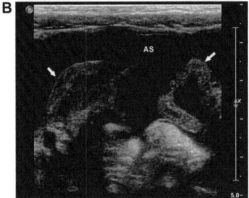

Fig. 21. (A) Sagittal image of the pelvis showing septated ascites with a latticelike appearance and a thickened greater omentum (arrow). (B) Transverse image showing bilateral irregularly thickened fallopian tubes (arrows) floating in the ascitic fluid (AS).

the combination of these features particularly with septated ascites is in favor of tuberculosis,[66,68] and laparoscopy and biopsy can be used to confirm the diagnosis. When a patient presents with infertility, ultrasonography may reveal a hydrosalpinx, but if no abnormality is seen, saline

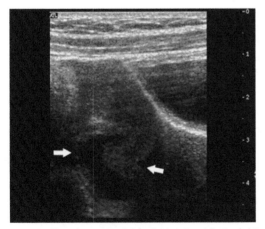

Fig. 22. The dry type of pelvic tuberculosis with a thick-walled fluid-distended fallopian tube (arrows).

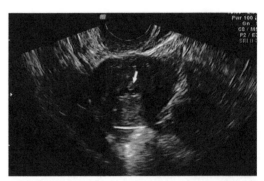

Fig. 23. Saline infusion sonohysterographic image showing an irregular endometrial contour with a polyp (arrow).

infusion sonohysterography may reveal either tubal block or abnormal fallopian tubes.

Endometrial tuberculosis

The uterine endometrium is involved in 50% of patients who have tubal tuberculosis.[62,69] It is involved by the extension of the disease from the fallopian tube and is seen in 11.5% of patients with pulmonary tuberculosis.[70] The pathology similarly involves the formation of granulomas and caseous necrosis resulting in a shrunken cavity as a result of adhesions and calcification. Patients present with infertility (45%–55%) and menstrual disturbances (20%) or amenorrhea, although some patients may be asymptomatic.[71] Saline infusion sonohysterography is the technique of choice used to reveal some of the features of endometrial tuberculosis, and the specific features that are suggestive of tuberculosis are irregular contour of the endometrium, endometrial polyps, synechiae, and a scarred cavity (Fig. 23). Endometrial calcification is seen as tiny specks of bright echoes in the endometrium (Fig. 24) and if extensive, can mimic endometrial osseous metaplasia. Dilation

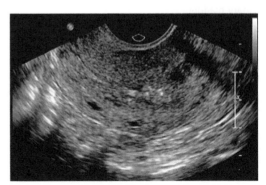

Fig. 24. Longitudinal image of the uterus showing punctate calcification in the endometrium.

and curettage or hysteroscopic biopsy has to be performed for histologic diagnosis.

ACKNOWLEDGMENTS

The author thanks Srambical Sreedharan, EDP, for technical assistance and Padma Ramesh for secretarial assistance in the preparation of this article. The author also thanks all the clinical colleagues for their cooperation.

REFERENCES

1. Kennedy DH. Extrapulmonary tuberculosis. In: Ratledge C, Stanford JL, Grange JM, editors. The biology of the mycobacteria, vol. III. New York: Academic Press; 1989. p. 245–84.

2. Kim SH. Genitourinary tuberculosis. In: Pollack HM, McClennan BL, editors. Clinical urography. 2nd edition. Philadelphia: WB Saunders Co; 2000. p. 1193–228.

3. Sharma SK, Mohan A. Extrapulmonary tuberculosis. Indian J Med Res 2004;120:316–53.

4. Heaton ND, Hogan B, Michell M, et al. Tuberculous epididymo-orchitis: clinical and ultrasound observations. Br J Urol 1989;64:305–9.

5. Premkumar A, Lattimer J, Newhouse JH. CT and sonography of advanced urinary tract tuberculosis. AJR Am J Roentgenol 1987;148:65–9.

6. Becker JA. Renal tuberculosis. Urol Radiol 1988;10: 25–30.

7. Mohan A, Sharma SK. Epidemiology. In: Sharma SK, Mohan A, editors. Tuberculosis. New Delhi (India): Jaypee Brothers Medical Publishers; 2001. p. 14–29.

8. Balasubramaniam R, Ramachandran R. Management of non-pulmonary forms of tuberculosis: review of TRC studies over two decades. Indian J Pediatr 2000;67:34–40.

9. Chaisson RE, Slutkin G. Tuberculosis and human immunodeficiency virus infection. J Infect Dis 1989;159:96–100.

10. Wolf JS Jr, McAninch JW. Tuberculous epididymo-orchitis: diagnosis by fine needle aspiration. J Urol 1991;145:836–8.

11. Cohen MS. Granulomatous nephritis. Urol Clin North Am 1986;13:647–59.

12. Kim SH, Kim SH, Kim WH. Imaging makes progress in urinary tract tuberculosis. Diagn Imaging Asia Pac 1995;2:22–8.

13. Goldman SM, Fishman EK, Hartman DS, et al. Computed tomography of renal tuberculosis and its pathological correlates. J Comput Assist Tomogr 1985;9:771–6.

14. Tonkin AK, Witten DM. Genitourinary tuberculosis. Semin Roentgenol 1979;14:305–18.

15. Eastwood JB, Dilly SA, GraElnge JM. Renal mycobacterial diseases. 4th edition. Philadelphia: Lippincott Williams & Wilkins; 2001.

16. Wise GJ, Marella VK. Genitourinary manifestations of tuberculosis. Urol Clin North Am 2003;30: 111–21.

17. Gupta NP, Kumar R, Mundada OP, et al. Reconstructive surgery for the management of genitourinary tuberculosis: a single center experience. J Urol 2006;175:2150–4.

18. Das KM, Vaidyanathan S, Rajwanshi A, et al. Renal tuberculosis: diagnosis with sonographically guided aspiration cytology. AJR Am J Roentgenol 1992;158: 571–3.

19. Schaffer R, Becker JA, Goodman J. Sonography of tuberculous kidney. Urology 1983;22:209–11.

20. Das KM, Indudhara R, Vaidyanathan S. Sonographic features of genitourinary tuberculosis. AJR Am J Roentgenol 1992;158:327–9.

21. Vijayaraghavan SB, Kandasamy SV, Arul M, et al. Spectrum of high-resolution sonographic features of urinary tuberculosis. J Ultrasound Med 2004;23: 585–94.

22. Elkin M. Urogenital tuberculosis. Philadelphia: WB Saunders Co; 1990.

23. Barrie HJ, Kerr WK, Gale GL. The incidence and pathogenesis of tuberculous strictures of the renal pyelus. J Urol 1967;98:584–9.

24. Gow JG. Renal calcification in genito-urinary tuberculosis. Br J Surg 1965;52:283–8.

25. McAleer SJ, Johnson CW, Johnson WD. Tuberculosis and parasitic and fungal infections of the genitourinary system. In: Wein AJ, Kavoussi LR, Novick AC, et al, editors. Campbell-Walsh urology. 9th edition. Philadelphia: WB Saunders; 2007. p. 436–70.

26. Sutherland AM, Glen ES, MacFarlane JR. Transmission of genito-urinary tuberculosis. Health Bull (Edinb) 1982;40:87–91.

27. Smith. General urology. 13th edition. California: Appleton and Lange; 1992. p. 240.

28. Auerbach O. Pathology of urogenital tuberculosis. New Intern Clin 1940;3:21.

29. Kumar R. Reproductive tract tuberculosis and male infertility. Indian J Urol 2008;24:392–5.

30. Kapoor R, Ansari MS, Mandhani A, et al. Clinical presentation and diagnostic approach in cases of genitourinary tuberculosis. Indian J Urol 2008;24:401–5.

31. Hamrick-Turner J, Abbitt PL, Ros PR. Tuberculosis of the lower genitourinary tract: findings on sonography and MR. AJR Am J Roentgenol 1992;158:919.

32. Wolf LE. Tuberculous abscess of the prostate in AIDS. Ann Intern Med 1996;125:156.

33. Tikkakoski T, Karstrup S, Lohela P, et al. Tuberculosis of the lower genitourinary tract: ultrasonography as an aid to diagnosis and treatment. J Clin Ultrasound 1993;21:269–71.

34. Riehle RA Jr, Jayaraman K. Tuberculosis of testis. Urology 1982;20:43–6.

35. Chung JJ, Kim MJ, Lee T, et al. Sonographic findings in tuberculous epididymitis and epididymo-orchitis. J Clin Ultrasound 1997;25:390–4.

36. Koyama Y, Iigaya T, Saito S. Tuberculous epididymo-orchitis. Urology 1988;31:419–21.

37. Gow JG. Genitourinary tuberculosis. Philadelphia: WB Saunders; 1986.

38. Smith DR. Specific infections of the urinary tract. 10th edition. Los Altos (CA): LMP; 1981.

39. Muttarak M, Lojanapiwat B, Chaiwun B, et al. Preoperative diagnosis of bilateral tuberculous epididymo-orchitis following intravesical Bacillus Calmette-Guerin therapy for superficial bladder carcinoma. Australas Radiol 2002;46:183–5.

40. Drudi FM, Laghi A, Iannicelli E, et al. Tubercular epididymitis and orchitis: US patterns. Eur Radiol 1997;7:1076–8.

41. Kim SH, Pollack HM, Cho KS, et al. Tuberculous epididymitis and epididymo-orchitis: sonographic findings. J Urol 1993;150:81–4.

42. Muttarak M, Peh WC, Lojanapiwat B, et al. Tuberculous epididymitis and epididymo-orchitis: sonographic appearances. AJR Am J Roentgenol 2001; 176:1459–66.

43. Turkvatan A, Kelahmet E, Yazgan C, et al. Sonographic findings in tuberculous epididymo-orchitis. J Clin Ultrasound 2004;32:302–5.

44. Ferrie BG, Rundle JS. Tuberculous epididymo-orchitis. A review of 20 cases. Br J Urol 1983;55: 437–9.

45. Ross JC, Gow JG, St Hill CA. Tuberculous epididymitis. A review of 170 patients. Br J Surg 1961;48: 663–6.

46. Mostofi FK, Davis CJJ. Male reproductive system and prostate. St Louis (MO): Mosby; 1990.

47. Reeve HR, Weinerth JL, Peterson LJ. Tuberculosis of epididymis and testicle presenting as hydrocele. Urology 1974;4:329–31.

48. Gorse GJ, Belshe RB. Male genital tuberculosis: a review of the literature with instructive case reports. Rev Infect Dis 1985;7:511–24.

49. Wechsler H, Westfall M, Lattimer JK. The earliest signs and symptoms in 127 male patients with genitourinary tuberculosis. J Urol 1960;83:801–3.

50. Barthwick WM. The pathogenesis of tuberculous epididymitis. Edinb Med J 1946;53:55.

51. Hill GS, Billey-kijner C. Paratesticular structures: nontumorous conditions. New York: Churchill Livingstone; 1989.

52. Yang DM, Chang MS, Oh YH, et al. Chronic tuberculous epididymitis: color Doppler US findings with histopathologic correlation. Abdom Imaging 2000; 25:559–62.

53. Yang DM, Yoon MH, Kim HS, et al. Comparison of tuberculous and pyogenic epididymal abscesses: clinical, gray-scale sonographic, and color Doppler sonographic features. AJR Am J Roentgenol 2001; 177:1131–5.

54. Kratzik C, Hainz A, Kuber W, et al. Sonographic appearance of benign intratesticular lesions. Eur Urol 1988;15:196–9.

55. Hamm B. Differential diagnosis of scrotal masses by ultrasound. Eur Radiol 1997;7:668–79.

56. Salmeron I, Ramirez-Escobar MA, Puertas F, et al. Granulomatous epididymo-orchitis: sonographic features and clinical outcome in brucellosis, tuberculosis, and idiopathic granulomatous epididymo-orchitis. J Urol 1998;159:1954–7.

57. Dempsey J, Brooks J, Scott RL. Testicular pseudotumor caused by Mycobacterium bovis epididymitis. J Clin Ultrasound 1992;20:200–3.

58. Estham JA, Spires KS, Abreo F. Seminal vesicle abscess due to tuberculosis: role of tissue culture in making the diagnosis. South Med J 1999;98:328.

59. Paick J, Kim SH, Kim SW. Ejaculatory duct obstruction in infertile men. Br J Urol 2000;85:720–4.

60. Kumar R, Thulkar S, Kumar V, et al. Contribution of investigations to the diagnosis of bilateral vas aplasia. ANZ J Surg 2005;75:807–9.

61. Pal DK. Tubercular abscess of the seminal vesicle. Ind J Tub 2003;50:155.

62. Siegler AM, Kontopoulos V. Female genital tuberculosis and the role of hysterosalpingography. Semin Roentgenol 1979;14:295–304.

63. Nogales-Ortiz F, Tarancon I, Nogales FF Jr. The pathology of female genital tuberculosis. A 31-year study of 1436 cases. Obstet Gynecol 1979;53: 422–8.

64. Yorder IC. Hysterosalpingography and pelvic ultrasound: imaging in infertility and gynecology. 1st edition. Boston: Little Brown and Company; 1988.

65. Merchant SA. Genital tract tuberculosis. 1st edition. New Delhi (India): Jaypee Brothers; 1997.

66. Yapar EG, Ekici E, Karasahin E, et al. Sonographic features of tuberculous peritonitis with female genital tract tuberculosis. Ultrasound Obstet Gynecol 1995; 6:121–5.

67. Thompson JD, Spence JD. Pelvic inflammatory disease. Philadelphia: J.B. Lippincott; 1992.

68. Tongsong T, Sukpan K, Wanapirak C, et al. Sonographic features of female pelvic tuberculous peritonitis. J Ultrasound Med 2007;26:77–82.

69. Premkumar A. Genitourinary tuberculosis and schistosomiasis. In: Taveras JM, Ferrucci JT, editors, In: Radiology-diagnosis-imaging-intervention, vol. 4. Philadelphia: J.B. Lippincott; 1986. p. 1–6.

70. Mukkerji VK, Misra J, Nath R, et al. A study of endometrial tuberculosis in hospitalised patients of pulmonary tuberculosis. Ind J Tub 1991;38:197–9.

71. Chowdhury NN. Overview of tuberculosis of the female genital tract. J Indian Med Assoc 1996;94: 345–6, 361.

Renal Transplant Assessment: Sonographic Imaging

Aneeta Parthipun, MBBS, FRCR,
James Pilcher, MBBS, MSc, MRCP, FRCR*

KEYWORDS

• Doppler studies • Renal transplantation • Ultrasonography

The first successful renal transplant was performed in 1954 between identical twins in the United States.[1] However it was not until the 1960s, with the introduction of immunosuppressive agents, that cadaveric and nonsibling transplantation became a realistic procedure.[2] Over the past 4 decades there has been marked improvement in the results of renal transplantation because of modifications in surgical technique, advances in preoperative tissue typing, new generations of immunosuppressive agents, and developments in graft preservation techniques, such as interventional radiology.[3,4]

Renal transplantation has transformed the treatment of end-stage renal disease and has been proven to be highly cost effective compared with long-term dialysis.[5] Not only does it deliver a major improvement in patient life quality by freeing the recipient from dialysis, but it also confers a significant survival benefit, with a calculated standardized mortality rate of 2.0/100 patient years for a live donor transplant compared with 6.3/100 patient years for dialysis. In the United States, the life expectancy for a patient 1 year after transplantation is 95% to 98%, whereas the current half-life for grafts from living donors is 21.6 years and from nonliving donors it is 13.8 years.[6] The major limiting factor in transplantation is now the relative lack of available donor organs. In response to this, the number of living donor transplants is increasing and kidneys that would have previously been deemed unsuitable because of complex vascular anatomy, atypical morphology (eg, horseshoe), or a non−heart beating donor are now being transplanted.[7]

Routine sonographic evaluation of renal transplants began in the 1970s, with the introduction of Doppler techniques 10 years later. Ultrasonography has become the main imaging modality in the initial assessment of graft dysfunction and may be used to guide subsequent interventional procedures.[8] It is also routinely used in the long-term follow-up of the transplant, where its role is one of surveillance for possible late-onset complications. Observer reproducibility is therefore essential if the examination is to carry any validity, which requires careful attention toward examination technique, along with a clear understanding by the operator of the normal gray-scale and color Doppler findings. Hence, this article aims to review both the scan technique and sonographic appearances of the normal renal transplant, while highlighting the role of this modality in various causes of graft dysfunction.

ULTRASOUND ANATOMY

Basic understanding of the surgical technique and the anatomy of the possible vascular anastomoses is very useful for the sonographer in both performing and interpreting the ultrasound examination. Usually the transplant kidney is positioned within the retroperitoneum in the right iliac fossa, with an end-to-side anastomosis of the renal vasculature to the recipient's external iliac artery and vein.[9,10] The left iliac fossa is used if there is vascular disease in the right iliac vessels, in second transplants, and in the case of combined renal and pancreas transplants.

Radiology Department, St George's Hospital, Blackshaw Road, London SW17 0QT, UK
* Corresponding author.
E-mail address: James.Pilcher@stgeorges.nhs.uk

Ultrasound Clin 5 (2010) 379–399
doi:10.1016/j.cult.2010.08.004
1556-858X/10/$ — see front matter © 2010 Elsevier Inc. All rights reserved.

The type of arterial anastomosis depends on whether the graft is from a live donor or a cadaveric graft. Cadaveric grafts are usually dissected with an intact main renal artery and a section of the aorta. The portion of the aorta is cut to an oval shape and then anastomosed, via an end-to-side technique, to the recipient's external iliac artery. With kidneys from living donors, a portion of the aorta obviously cannot be resected and therefore either an end-to-side anastomosis of the donor renal artery to the recipient's external iliac artery or an end-to-end anastomosis to the internal iliac artery is performed. The donor vein is sutured in an end-to-side anastomosis to the external iliac vein. Multiple arterial or venous anastomoses are required in approximately 20% of renal transplants and in these situations good surgical documentation of the procedure, ideally with an illustration of the procedure, can prove invaluable to the operator. The transplant ureter is anastomosed to the superior aspect of the bladder using a technique known as an extravesical ureteroneocystostomy, whereby the ureter is effectively tunneled through the detrusor muscle and sutured to the bladder mucosa.[11] A ureteric stent is often initially left in situ to avoid early ureteric complications, being removed somewhere between 2 weeks and 3 months.[12]

SONOGRAPHIC TECHNIQUE

A successful comprehensive sonographic examination of the transplant kidney requires a careful systematic approach and equipment that offers excellent Doppler sensitivity, being able to perform high pulse repetition frequency (PRF) sampling to a reasonable depth. Because of the relatively superficial position of the transplant, it is often possible to use a curvilinear array with a central frequency of around 6 MHz, although in the immediate postoperative assessment this may need to be reduced owing to soft tissue induration and fluid collections around the transplant. Before commencing the examination, the operator should ideally have reviewed any previous imaging of the transplant, have access to the surgical record for the vascular anatomy of the transplant, and be aware of any potentially complicating factors such as prolonged ischemia times.

The orientation of the transplant within the pelvis is highly variable and therefore there is no set approach to obtaining standard longitudinal and transverse views of the graft. A coronal plane is also usually attainable, which affords a good view of the renal hilum, helping to determine the course of the pelvicalyceal system and feeding vessels. Gray-scale assessment of the transplant

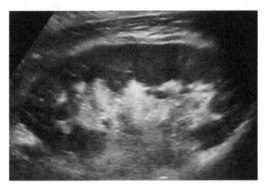

Fig. 1. A normal transplant kidney, demonstrating good contrast resolution between cortex and medulla. The echogenic sinus fat is split by vessels and collecting system.

includes the identification of any fluid collections adjacent or superficial to the transplant. The length and volume of the graft may be recorded, although this does suffer from significant interobserver error and is of limited value.[13] As a result of the graft's superficial position, the contrast in relative reflectivity between the cortex, medullary pyramids, and sinus fat is far more apparent than in native kidneys (**Fig. 1**). The collecting system is also assessed for any hydronephrosis or ureteric dilatation.

A rapid assessment of global transplant perfusion can then be made by adjusting the color box volume to incorporate the whole graft, while optimizing the PRF and color gain. In the immediate postoperative transplant, the Doppler signal toward the periphery of the polar aspects of the graft is often poor, in part because of the angle of insonation. If it is not possible to reposition the probe, because of surgical dressings, power Doppler can be useful in confirming flow in these

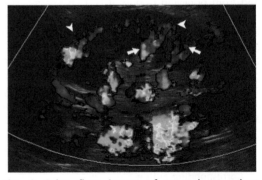

Fig. 2. Color flow image of normal transplant, demonstrating interlobar and arcuate vessels (*arrows*) and the peripheral cortical branches (*arrowheads*).

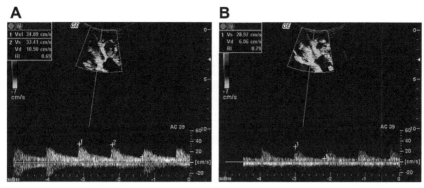

Fig. 3. (*A*) An RI measurement taken from an arcuate vessel with light probe pressure. (*B*) By increasing the probe pressure over the transplant the measured RI has significantly increased from 0.69 to 0.79.

areas.[14] The sample volume is then reduced to allow for a more targeted assessment of the interlobular or arcuate vessels using spectral Doppler: the more peripheral interlobular vessels should be avoided because of increasing inter- and intraobserver variability (**Fig. 2**).[15] The most common Doppler indices used to assess the blood flow within the graft are the pulsatility index (PI), resistive index (RI), and the acceleration time (AT). Which of these, if any, are used will partly depend on local protocol and partly on the appearance of the spectral Doppler trace at the time of scanning. At least 3 areas of the graft should be assessed in this way, typically the upper, lower, and interpolar regions. Care must be taken regarding the degree of pressure applied with the probe over the transplant, as the parenchyma can be easily compressed resulting in reduced diastolic inflow (**Fig. 3**).[16]

The main transplant artery (or arteries) and vein are then assessed, using color Doppler to trace each of them back from the renal hilum to their respective anastomoses. This can often be challenging because of the tortuous pathway taken by some vessels as a result of surgical technique. Angle-corrected (<60°) spectral Doppler traces should then be recorded at each arterial anastomosis and at any point along the artery, where there is color aliasing suggesting high-velocity flow (**Fig. 4**).[17] In the immediate postoperative period this may not be possible because of surrounding tissue edema and limited access from dressings and drains. The patency of the transplant vein is also confirmed with both color and spectral Doppler. Formal spectral Doppler interrogation of the iliac vessels is not routinely necessary unless there is concern over an anastomotic stricture or more unusually a stenosis of the iliac vessel itself (**Fig. 5**). The bladder should also be routinely scanned to confirm the position of

any stent in situ and to rule out the presence of echogenic debris that may be secondary to hemorrhage or infection.

For each patient, the timing and frequency of successive sonographic examinations will be determined by a combination of local protocol and the current clinical and laboratory findings. At our institution, we perform an immediate postoperative examination on every patient in recovery; with further examinations during their in-patient stay determined by these sonographic findings and their subsequent clinical picture. A 6-week examination is performed following removal of the ureteric stent, following which the patient enters a program of annual routine follow-up examinations, unless there is a transplant-related clinical episode.

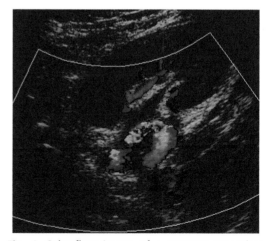

Fig. 4. Color-flow image of a tortuous transplant artery showing a number of areas where there is color aliasing; all of these will require interrogation with angle-corrected spectral Doppler.

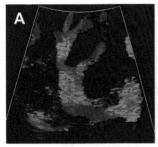
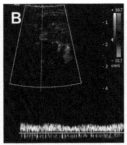
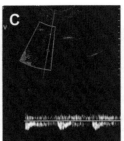
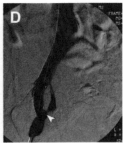

Fig. 5. (*A*) A 5-month old poorly functioning renal transplant, with color flow imaging at the renal hilum showing complete reversal of flow in a rather distended transplant vein. (*B*) A close-up view of transplant cortex shows multiple venous collaterals crossing the cortex extending out into the retroperitoneum. (*C*) The external iliac vein demonstrates pulsatile venous flow and the common iliac vein could not be demonstrated. A subsequent venous angiogram showed complete occlusion of common iliac and proximal external iliac vein with venous return from the lower limb diverted through the transplant vein. (*D*) The iliac vein was successfully recannulated and a stent placed across the underlying stenosis just proximal to the origin of the transplant vein (*arrowhead*).

THE NORMAL TRANSPLANT

The normal transplant kidney has the same sonographic features as a native kidney, although the parenchymal detail is typically much clearer. The renal cortex makes up most of the renal tissue, forming an outer peripheral rim of mid-gray echoes that surround the relatively echo-poor medullary pyramids. Each pyramid is also encased by the interlobular cortical tissue that extends down to the renal sinus, the latter being highly reflective owing to its variable fat content and vascular interfaces (see **Fig. 1**). The collecting system is often partly visible, particularly in the new transplant because of edema at the vesicoureteric anastomosis. Making the distinction between significant dilatation can therefore sometimes be difficult, although filling of the infundibulum and calyces should be treated with suspicion (**Fig. 6**). The proximal ureter can often be identified, but then quickly tapers, becoming difficult to visualize unless a ureteric stent is in situ.

If measured, the renal dimensions are similar to that of a native adult kidney and in the new transplant a gradual increase in these dimensions is seen over the first few weeks by up to 32% of the initial length by the fourth week.[18] With optimized color Doppler settings, flow can be demonstrated out to the cortical branches of the interlobular vessels (see **Fig. 2**); toward the renal poles, power Doppler may be required to show this. The normal spectral trace obtained from the interlobar vessels shows a "low-resistance" pattern with continuous forward flow throughout the cardiac cycle. A sharp systolic upstroke is followed by a slow diastolic decay (described as a "ski-slope" appearance), with the diastolic velocity remaining between one-third to one-half

that of the peak systolic velocity (PSV)[19] (**Fig. 7**). A reduction in diastolic flow may indicate underlying pathology. The main transplant artery demonstrates a similar low-resistance waveform with angle-corrected velocities measuring somewhere around 100 cm/s. The spectral Doppler trace from the main transplant vein is often quite pulsatile in nature and this is partly because of systolic compression from the adjacent artery.

THE RESISTIVE INDEX AND ACCELERATION TIME

The RI is a frequently used parameter in transplant Doppler, measuring the ratio of end diastolic flow to peak systolic flow within the transplant. Initially there was great enthusiasm for the RI in transplant ultrasound, as it was thought to be highly specific in the diagnosis of acute rejection[20]; however,

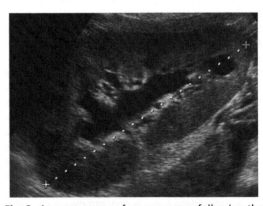

Fig. 6. An appearance of some concern following the removal of a ureteric stent, with dilatation of collecting system extending out to the calyces, in a patient with an empty bladder.

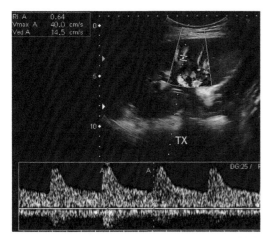

Fig. 7. Acquisition of interpolar RI value, with the spectral gate placed over an interlobar artery; as this is a ratio measurement, angle correction is not critical. The spectral trace shows good anterior flow throughout diastole.

subsequent studies have failed to support this.[21,22] Although it is still used in many centers, interpretation should be limited to serial changes in its value acting as a marker of transplant dysfunction. This approach mirrors an increased understanding of the factors that affect the renal arterial Doppler waveform.[23] Although renal vascular resistance does have some influence on the RI measurement, there is now good evidence demonstrating a strong dependence on the vascular compliance and the pulse pressure of the recipient's central arterial circulation.[24] In line with this, the recipient's age and cardiovascular risk factors have also been shown to correlate with changes in RI measurement.[24,25] Therefore, interpretation of an elevated RI needs to be taken in the context of these factors, along with any clinical and biochemical findings. The normal value for the RI is about 0.60, with the upper limit of normal being 0.70.

The pulsatility index is used by some centers as an alternative measure of vascular impedance within the interlobar arteries with a value greater than 1.8 being seen as significantly elevated. The acceleration time is usually measured from spectral Doppler traces in the segmental arteries and is the time between the start of systole and the first systolic peak. The normal quoted value is 70 ms or less and values above this are indicative of upstream disease; namely, a stenosis in the main artery or at the anastomosis. Other investigators have proposed setting a higher value of 80 ms or more[26] to increase its specificity. There has also been some interest in the use of the AT index for the prediction of acute graft dysfunction in the first day after transplantation, where a value of less

than 90 ms has been used.[27] Other groups have shown an association between cyclosporin A toxicity and a prolonged acceleration time, although this was statistically unreliable.[28]

TRANSPLANT COMPLICATIONS

Improvements in surgical technique and use of potent immunosuppressive agents has seen a significant reduction in early complication rates and increasingly the focus of patient follow-up is on preventing later complications. Clinically, the presentation of most transplant complications is rather nonspecific, with the possibility of poorly controlled hypertension, diminishing urine output, rising serum creatinine, elevated inflammatory markers, pain over the transplant site, and fever. Early diagnosis of the underlying cause of transplant dysfunction is vital to ensure optimal management and preservation of the graft. Ultrasonography plays a central role in the detection, management, and follow-up of both early and late complications, which can be divided into the categories described in the following sections.

Parenchymal Complications

Delayed graft function is a common occurrence following transplantation, which in the cadaveric transplant is often because of acute tubular necrosis (ATN), with the main differentials being acute rejection and immunosuppressive drug toxicity. As these all require quite different management strategies, accurate distinction between them is essential and this often requires histology. Although a number of early studies described gray-scale and Doppler sonographic features that could reliably distinguish rejection from ATN, later work has failed to substantiate this. Despite this failing, ultrasonography still has an important role to play in the early monitoring of graft function, providing an initial qualitative assessment of graft perfusion and subsequently through serial RI or PI measurements of the interlobar vessels. In conjunction with clinical and biochemical findings, the latter can be used to monitor any emerging graft dysfunction and assist in guiding the clinician as to the need to biopsy. The subsequent response to any alteration in therapy can also be assessed through serial Doppler measurements.

Acute Tubular Necrosis

Acute tubular necrosis is initially present in most cadaveric transplants, usually resolving over a period of 1 to 2 weeks, although it can occasionally last up to 3 months. Dialysis support may be required in up to 20% of cases, which may be antagonized by the use of certain immunosuppressive agents. The underlying cause is attributable to a combination of cold ischemia and reperfusion injury and is particularly prominent in the non–heart beating donor kidney. It is relatively unusual in live donor kidneys unless there is a surgical complication during implantation. Even upon recovery there may be long-term compromise to graft survival, with the very process of tubular cell repair increasing the risk of acute rejection.[29]

The sonographic appearances are nonspecific, with some swelling of the graft on gray-scale imaging, leading to a slight increase in graft length, and reduced diastolic flow (elevated RI or PI) in the interlobar vessels (**Fig. 8**). Sometimes this can be so marked that the direction of flow drops below the baseline in diastole[30]; this may even be seen in the immediate postoperative period. In one perioperative study, an RI of greater than 0.73 in the hilar area of the main artery 30 minutes after unclamping iliac vessels was strongly predictive for subsequent ATN.[31] If radionuclide imaging is used, it will demonstrate a delayed transit time and time to maximal activity followed by impaired secretion of isotope, with increasing parenchymal retention of isotope on sequential images.

Acute Rejection

With the use of modern immunosuppressive agents such as the calcineurin inhibitors, the incidence of acute rejection has significantly reduced over the past decade. It is now happens in about 20% of all transplants and occurs within the first 6 months following surgery. Despite effective management with high-dose steroids and immunosuppressive medication, an episode of rejection still carries a significant adverse prognostic outlook for long-term graft survival.[32] The patient is often asymptomatic, but can present with low-grade pyrexia and graft tenderness.

Previously described associated gray scale features include marked parenchymal swelling (typically more than seen with ATN), with compression of the sinus fat, increased prominence of the renal pyramids, and thickening of the collecting system urothelium,[33] all of which have subsequently been shown to be completely nonspecific (**Fig. 9**). Likewise, the use of Doppler to identify elevated RIs within the interlobar vessels has now been shown to be a nonspecific finding (**Table 1**) and in the mild to moderate stages of rejection the RI is often normal. Serial examinations and measurement of the RI is useful in cases of rejection, primarily as an indicator of when to biopsy the graft, but also in monitoring its recovery following appropriate immunosuppression. Previously there was an interest in using power Doppler to demonstrate pruning of the peripheral intrarenal arteries as a sign of acute rejection, but as with the gray-scale findings, this has subsequently been shown to be a nonspecific finding.[34]

Calcineurin Inhibitor Nephrotoxicity

The calcineurin inhibitors cyclosporin and tacrolimus have been key immunosuppressive agents in the success of renal transplantation with regard to the management of rejection. Unfortunately they are also nephrotoxic, causing renovascular constriction and with long-term use interstitial fibrosis.[35] In addition, polyomavirus-associated nephropathy (PAN) is a recently described condition linked with these agents, believed to be a latent virus reactivated by immunosuppressive damage at a tubular level. The resulting clinical

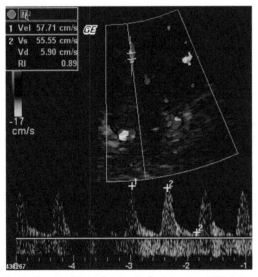

Fig. 8. Spectral Doppler study from an arcuate artery in a patient with acute tubular necrosis, showing a significant reduction in end diastolic blood flow.

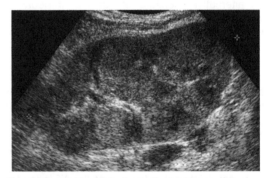

Fig. 9. Grossly swollen transplant kidney with sinus fat compression and loss of normal cortical medullary differentiation in a patient with acute rejection.

Table 1
Causes of an elevated resistive index value in the interlobar arteries

Causes of Elevated Resistive Index	
Parenchymal	Acute rejection
	Acute tubular necrosis
	Pyelonephritis
Vascular	Renal vein thrombosis
	Hypotension
Urological	Ureteral obstruction
Technical	Graft compression
Physiologic	Bradycardia

picture is completely indistinguishable from chronic rejection.[36] Even with biopsy and serum drug levels, diagnosis and management of calcineurin toxicity and PAN can be very challenging. Neither of these conditions alters the RI values with any degree of reliability, and even in cases where it does, it cannot be distinguished from rejection or ATN.[37]

Infection

In the first 6 months, patients are at increased risk of infection because of their immunocompromised state, which can also mask the clinical presentation of a pyelonephritis.[38] Long-term, repeated infections can result in structural abnormalities, such as obstruction, reflux, and stone formation. As with the native kidney, the appearance of transplant infections on ultrasonography is variable and often nonspecific. Both urothelial thickening and focal or diffuse areas of low reflective parenchymal swelling are recognized findings, but these overlap significantly with rejection in the early stages. In a dilated collecting system, low-level echo content is highly suggestive of a pyonephrosis (**Fig. 10**), although this can appear anechoic. Focal rounded, nonshadowing, echogenic structures within the collecting system are highly suggestive of fungal balls.[39] Papillary necrosis can also occur as a result of certain infections, which in turn may lead to ureteric obstruction. Ultrasonography cannot reliably diagnose papillary necrosis (although cystic spaces in the renal pyramids have been described), which requires pyelography[11] or delayed contrast CT.

Chronic Allograft Nephropathy

Next to death of the recipient, chronic allograft nephropathy (CAN) is the main cause of long-term graft loss after the first year of transplant.[40,41] The etiology and pathogenesis of CAN is complex, with numerous contributing factors, including

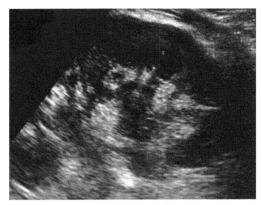

Fig. 10. Mild dilatation of the collecting system with moderate echogenic content, in a recent transplant patient with low-grade pyrexia and minimally elevated inflammatory markers.

previous episodes of acute rejection, subclinical rejection, delayed graft function, donor age, and calcineurin toxicity. Biopsies from a transplant with CAN show an overall fibrotic picture affecting the vascular endothelium, tubules, glomeruli, and interstitium. Clinically there is progressive deterioration in graft function, with proteinuria and hypertension.

Described ultrasound features of CAN include loss of graft volume, cortical thinning, and increased cortical reflectivity (**Fig. 11**). On color Doppler there tends to be a reduced number of visible intrarenal vessels, with straightening of the remaining vessels.[42] None of these findings are reliable in confirming the diagnosis of CAN, and the role of ultrasound is currently to exclude other causes of graft dysfunction and guide any transplant biopsy. There are a number of Doppler studies that have shown that having an interlobar RI of greater than 0.7 at 1 to 3 months after transplantation is associated with a poor prognostic outcome with respect to CAN.[43,44] There is now

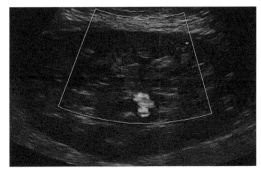

Fig. 11. Ten-year old transplant with gradually deteriorating renal function, showing reduced vascularity and some early cortical thinning, consistent with probable CAN.

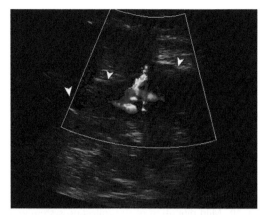

Fig. 12. Color flow imaging demonstrating active bleeding from a transplant arcuate vessel post biopsy: color flow is seen to extend beyond the margin of the cortex (*arrowheads*) into an accumulating hematoma.

increasing interest in the use of ultrasound microbubble contrast agents and elastography to detect CAN as early as possible.

GUIDED RENAL BIOPSY

In a significant number of delayed graft functions, biopsy is required to determine the underlying cause and ultrasonography is ideal for guiding this. The quoted complication rate for this procedure is about 5%[45] for perirenal hematomas (**Fig. 12**), arteriovenous fistula, hematuria, and a failed adequate sample. The use of ultrasonography helps avoid the major segmental vessels within the transplant and allows the needle to be positioned to maximize the core within the renal cortex rather than the medulla, the latter being associated with inadequate

sampling and an increased complication rate. Patel and colleagues[46] recently described a cortical tangential approach attempting to parallel the needle to the anterior cortical surface while scanning the transplant in either transverse or oblique sagittal planes. This resulted in a high-yield core enabling a reduction in needle caliber from 16G down to 18G.[46]

PERITRANSPLANT FLUID COLLECTION

In the immediate postsurgical period, small crescentic, echo-poor, fluid collections adjacent to the transplant are almost an expected finding and most likely represent small hematomas or seromas. For most of these no action is required, although it is good practice to document their size at the initial scan for monitoring purposes. Larger collections may cause problems through pressure effects on the collecting system, vascular pedicle, or bladder, requiring some form of intervention. The etiology of these collections is often difficult to determine solely on their sonographic appearance, but they usually represent a hematoma, urinoma, lymphocele, or less commonly an abscess. Changes in size and the timing of their appearance after transplant can help differentiate between these sonographically similar-appearing collections (**Table 2**).

Hematoma

Hematomas are relatively common in the immediate posttransplant period and are usually found within the subcutaneous tissues or around the transplant, with most resolving spontaneously. At

Table 2
Summary of timing and features of peritransplant fluid collections

Type	Timing Post Transplant	Sonographic Features	Incidence
Hematoma	Immediate	Echogenic with ill-defined margins. Becomes more defined with central cystic change ± fibrinous stranding.	Common
Abscess	Any time	Similar to hematoma Echogenic gas locules Color flow in surrounding tissue	Usually a consequence of an infected hematoma
Urinoma	Immediate	Anechoic Well defined Changes in size	Uncommon (1%–6%)
Lymphocele	4–8 weeks	Anechoic ± septations Typically between the bladder and transplant or along the medial aspect of the transplant	Common

ultrasonography, acute hematomas appear relatively echogenic and solid, but with time will liquefy, becoming more defined and cystic, often containing echogenic fibrinous septations and adherent clot debris. Percutaneous aspiration or drainage of these small collections is not advisable owing to their self-limiting nature and the risk of introducing infection. Larger hematomas can compromise the collecting system (**Fig. 13**) or vascular supply of the transplant, necessitating percutaneous drainage under sonographic guidance,[47] although if loculated, their complete drainage may not always be possible. Hematomas can also occur posttransplant biopsy (see **Fig. 13**) or following an interventional procedure, when they may be subcapsular in location (**Fig. 14**), appearing as a relatively low-reflective avascular area conforming to the renal contour. This can lead to an acute deterioration in renal function with loss of diastolic flow on spectral Doppler, requiring urgent percutaneous or surgical drainage.[48]

Abscess

Superadded infection of any of the peritransplant collections may result in abscess formation, which can be difficult to distinguish from a hematoma. In addition, clinical features of infection are often masked owing to immunosuppression. The typical sonographic findings of a fluid collection with low-level echoes and an irregular wall are seen in only a small percentage of cases. Power or color Doppler may be helpful by detecting increased vascularity in the surrounding tissues[42] and there is almost certainly a role for contrast ultrasound in confirming the inflammatory nature of such a collection. In the pyrexial patient, a perinephric collection should therefore be presumed to be

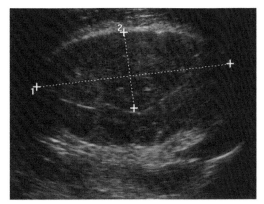

Fig. 14. Subcapsular hematoma following transplant artery stenting (*between cursors*). This was significantly distorting the transplant, compromising arterial inflow and required urgent percutaneous drainage.

infected until proven otherwise through the appropriate imaging and guided diagnostic aspiration. If confirmed, ultrasonography can be used to guide any percutaneous drainage that is required.

Urinoma

Occurring in only 1% to 6% of transplants,[49] these collections usually develop early, either as a result of extravasation at the ureterovesical anastomosis or from distal ureteral necrosis secondary to ischemia (**Fig. 15**). As a result, they tend to form close to the bladder, but can on occasion be found in unusual locations such as the scrotum or proximal thigh. Large urinomas may rupture into the peritoneum to cause a sterile peritonitis.[50] At ultrasonography, urinomas are almost always well defined, anechoic with no septations, and can change in size rapidly. A cystogram or isotope renography with delayed images may be helpful in confirming the urinary leak.

Lymphocele

Lymphoceles occur owing to disruption of the lymphatics along the iliac vessels or around the hilum of the transplanted kidney. These tend develop 1 to 2 months after transplantation, and can affect up to 20% of patients.[51] Usually an incidental finding, they are typically anechoic, but may contain septa and are typically positioned between the bladder and the medial aspect of the transplant. Although most simply require monitoring, lymphoceles are the most common fluid collection to cause pressure effects on the collecting system of the transplant resulting in hydronephrosis. They may also compress the vascular pedicle of the transplant (**Fig. 16**) or the iliac

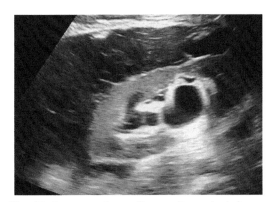

Fig. 13. Large postoperative peritransplant hematoma, probably causing some ureteric obstruction. The echotexture is very suggestive of hematoma, with mixed areas of reflectivity and evidence of early cystic change.

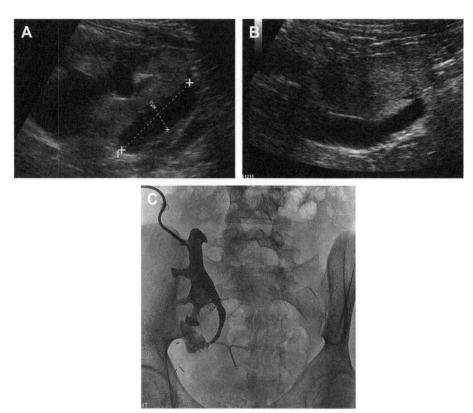

Fig. 15. (*A*) Focused view of the lower pole of a 1-year-old poorly functioning transplant, showing a small fluid collection that had appeared since the previous examination. Note the moderate hydronephrosis in the lower pole collecting system. (*B*) Focused view at the renal hilum showing dilated proximal ureter, with an abrupt apparent "cutoff" adjacent to the small fluid collection (not shown). (*C*) Subsequent nephrostomy for hydronephrosis confirms urine leak from mid-third of ureter, presumed to be ischemic in etiology.

vessels of the recipient, resulting in lower limb edema. In these situations, percutaneous drainage is required, with the fluid obtained demonstrating a creatinine level equal to that of serum. Lymphoceles often recur after percutaneous drainage, and the subsequent treatment options are either prolonged percutaneous catheter drainage with the installation of sclerosing agents, such as povidine-iodine, or laparoscopic marsupialization. Both techniques are reported to have a high success rate, although the size of the lymphocele may influence the choice of procedure.[52]

VASCULAR COMPLICATIONS

Vascular complications occur in fewer than 10% of transplant recipients, but are an important cause of graft dysfunction. Fortunately, most complications can now be managed by radiological intervention rather than surgery. Color and spectral Doppler ultrasonography are excellent at identifying most arterial and venous complications, although knowledge of the surgical anatomy is crucial for correct interpretation of the findings. Where there is uncertainty, conventional angiography or increasingly MR angiography is used to further characterize an abnormality.

Renal Artery Thrombosis

Thrombosis of the main renal artery is a rare (<1%) early complication that is usually attributable to a technical complication.[53] Contributing factors include multiple (therefore small) renal arteries, underlying atheromatous disease, pediatric donor kidney, and prolonged ischemic times. Color flow imaging of the transplant shows complete loss of any arterial or venous flow: it is important to ensure that the Doppler settings have been optimized for minimal flow. Spectral Doppler may demonstrate an attenuated systolic waveform in the proximal renal artery, with no diastolic flow. A similar finding may be seen in hyperacute rejection with microvascular thrombosis, although color flow still tends to be seen within the main renal artery in the latter, typically with reversed diastolic flow on spectral Doppler.[54] A flow pattern in the main transplant

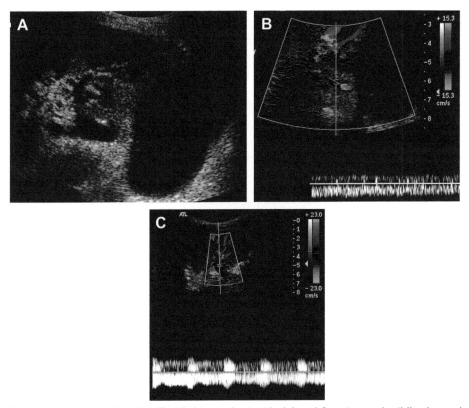

Fig. 16. Compressive lymphocele. (*A*) Left-sided transplant with delayed function and mildly elevated resistive indices on spectral Doppler, showing a moderately large lymphocele directly adjacent to the lower pole, with mild dilatation of the renal pelvis. (*B*) Duplex imaging of main transplant vein shows a small-caliber vessel, with a weak spectral Doppler trace. (*C*) Ultrasound-guided aspiration of lymphocele (400 mL) resulted in a significant increase in venous flow in the main transplant vein and reduction in the resistive indices back to normal values, with a subsequent improvement in renal function.

vein reflecting the cardiac cycle has also been described in hyperacute rejection owing to transmitted pressure changes from the inferior vena cava. In a transplant with multiple donor arteries, thrombosis of a single vessel will result in a segmental infarct, producing a focal, typically wedge-shaped area of low reflective swelling, with absence of any color flow (**Fig. 17**). Over time, this area will atrophy and become more reflective, forming a localized scar. Although a main artery thrombosis usually results in nephrectomy, there has been some reported success with graft fibrinolysis; likewise with recanalization of accessory branches.[55]

Renal Artery Stenosis

Transplant artery stenosis (TAS) is the most common vascular complication (up to 10%) seen within the first 3 months of transplantation. It can affect the iliac artery just proximal to the anastomosis (a surgical clamping injury), the anastomosis itself (owing to surgical technique), or the proximal renal artery (as a result of intimal ischemia). It is 3 times more likely to occur with an end-to-end anastomosis than an end-to side anastomosis.[56] Deteriorating renal function and severe resistant hypertension are suggestive clinical features. The relatively superficial position of the transplant vessels lends itself well toward the use of Doppler methods in reliably identifying a significant arterial stenosis, although it can be technically challenging if the artery has a particularly tortuous course. In these cases, power Doppler should be helpful in defining the pathway of the artery, but it will not highlight areas of disturbed flow. In addition, sharp bends or kinks in the artery can result in focal areas of color aliasing with increased velocity measurements that can mimic a stenosis. An angle-corrected peak systolic velocity (PSV) measurement of 200 to 250 cm/s is taken to indicate a significant stenosis,[26] although in the asymptomatic patient it has been suggested that a higher cutoff value be adopted of 300 cm/s.[57]

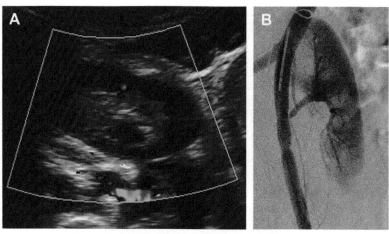

Fig. 17. (*A*) Transverse section through the lower pole of a new transplant, with a known small accessory artery showing reduced corticomedullary differentiation and absence of any color flow despite optimization of parameters. (*B*) Diagnostic angiogram confirms a lower pole segmental infarction, but it was not possible to recanalize the accessory vessel.

The PSV ratio between the prestenotic artery (often external iliac) and the stenotic segment should be greater than 2. The spectral trace just downstream of a stenosis will demonstrate spectral broadening reflecting the turbulent flow emerging from a tight stenosis (**Fig. 18**).

Within the segmental branches of the transplant, as with the native kidney, the finding of a tardus parvus waveform is often seen as an indirect sign of a significant proximal arterial stenosis. The Doppler indices used to define this waveform include an AT of more than 0.07 seconds and an AI of less than 300 cm/s^2; some units use an AT of 90 ms to increase specificity.[13] This slow-rising attenuated waveform also tends to result in a reduced RI measurement in the interlobar branches of less than 0.55, which may be the first finding that alerts the operator to a possible inflow problem. When both the direct and indirect Doppler measurements are combined, the overall accuracy for detecting TAS is as high as 95%.[58] MR angiography is now increasingly used, as opposed to conventional angiography, in cases where there remains uncertainty of the Doppler findings or there is a discrepancy between them and the clinical picture.

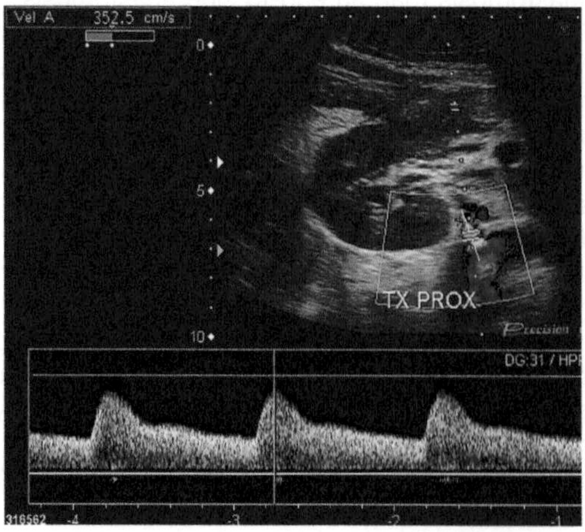

Stenosis of the iliac artery proximal to the anastomosis is relatively unusual, but should be suspected in a patient with an intrarenal tardus parvus waveform and no velocity rise in the main renal artery. These patients are likely to demonstrate loss of the normal triphasic waveform in the external iliac artery distal to the transplant artery anastomosis. A stenosis within a branch renal artery can be difficult to identify and occurs in chronic rejection or with parenchymal scarring following renal biopsy. There is regional altered blood flow on color flow imaging, and occasionally an intrarenal area of high-velocity flow is identified as a focus of color aliasing.

Renal Vein Thrombosis

Renal vein thrombosis is a relatively rare complication of transplantation but often results in early loss of the graft. It is more likely to occur following surgical difficulty with the venous anastomosis, episodes of hypovolemia, or if there is venous

Fig. 18. Significant renal artery stenosis just distal to the transplant artery anastomosis, with elevated peak systolic velocities and spectral broadening.

compression by a peritransplant collection. Typically, there is acute onset of oliguria, with swelling and tenderness over the graft site. Gray-scale appearances may demonstrate reduced corticomedullary differentiation, whereas color Doppler imaging shows arterial flow only during systole and sometimes intermittent color reversal in diastole; the use of power Doppler alone in these situations can therefore be highly misleading. The spectral Doppler waveform from the intrarenal arteries frequently shows striking reversal of flow throughout diastole, sometimes with an inverted "M" pattern (**Fig. 19**).[59] The combination of this finding with absence of a venous trace at the hilum is diagnostic for this condition and early recognition of this pattern is crucial for any chance of graft salvage through emergency thrombectomy. It should be remembered, however, that venous thrombosis initially occurs in the venules of the transplant so that sluggish flow may still be seen in the segmental veins early on in the process. Diastolic flow reversal can sometimes be seen in severe ATN or acute rejection (**Table 3**). Although it has been suggested that the flow reversal pattern in these other conditions tends only to occur at the beginning of diastole, this remains contentious.[30] A low-amplitude parvus-tardus arterial trace has also been reported in a few cases of venous thrombosis where there is incomplete venous occlusion.[60]

Table 3	
Causes of reverse diastolic flow.	
Perioperative Period	**Long Term (>30days)**
Severe acute tubular necrosis	Rejection
Acute rejection	Glomerulosclerosis
Renal vein thrombosis	Poor cardiac output
Compressive hematoma	
Graft torsion/kinked vessel	

Transplant Vein Stenosis

A localized stenosis of the main transplant vein is relatively unusual, but can occur anywhere along its length. Causes include compression by a perinephric fluid collection or trauma to the vein during surgery. Rather than an absolute value, the diagnosis requires a significant velocity gradient across the region of narrowing, ie, a three- to fourfold rise (**Fig. 20**).

Arteriovenous Fistulae and Pseudoaneurysms

Arteriovenous fistulae (AVF) are a well-recognized complication of renal transplant biopsy, with a reported incidence of up to 16% in biopsy series.[61] In general, most AVF are small and most (75%) will have spontaneously thrombosed by 4 weeks. On color Doppler they have a characteristic appearance, with a focus of intense color aliasing at the fistula site (**Fig. 21**). This can be highlighted by increasing the PRF until the normal intrarenal vessels are no longer visualized, leaving the feeding artery, nidus, and draining vein. Sometimes a flame-shaped band of color is seen to extend away from the AVF nidus, believed to represent tissue vibration as a result of the turbulent flow within the shunt. Spectral Doppler interrogation of the nidus will reveal a high-velocity low-resistance trace with marked spectral broadening, whereas an arterialized venous waveform is found in the draining vein. AVF have no hemodynamic consequence and are simply observed, but occasionally they can bleed or increase in size to cause a "steal phenomenon" requiring radiological embolization.[62]

A pseudoaneurysm (PA) is a far less common complication following biopsy (6%) and appears as a rounded cystic structure on gray-scale ultrasound. Color Doppler shows a characteristic overlapping red and blue pattern of turbulent flow within the PA sac (**Fig. 22**), whereas a characteristic to-and-fro waveform is seen on spectral

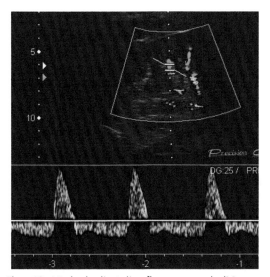

Fig. 19. Marked diastolic flow reversal (M-wave pattern) in a segmental artery seen in a graft with no detectable venous flow on optimized color or spectral Doppler. Although extremely sluggish flow was seen on gray-scale imaging in the segmental vessels, this is a recognized finding in evolving renal vein thrombosis.

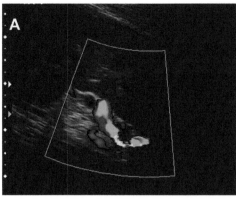
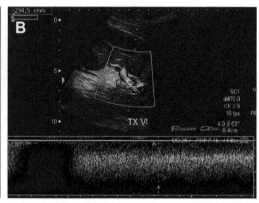

Fig. 20. (A) Color flow imaging study of a live donor kidney with mild renal impairment and slightly elevated resistive indices in the interlobar arteries. The main transplant vein shows a marked change in caliber and color aliasing as it passes between the 2 main transplant arteries at the level of the renal hilum. (B) Spectral Doppler interrogation of this segment showed a ×4 elevation in velocity consistent with a significant venous stenosis, presumably owing to compression by the 2 arteries.

Doppler at the neck of the PA. Again, most of these will thrombose spontaneously, but embolization should be considered if there is a significant increase in size (>2 cm).

Extrarenal pseudoaneurysms are extremely uncommon and tend to occur at the site of the arterial anastomosis as a result of surgical technique or infection. They are potentially devastating because of the high rupture risk and may present as a pulsating mass over the transplant site. Color Doppler will easily identify the PA, which has identical features to those described previously.[63]

UROLOGICAL COMPLICATIONS

Early ureteric obstruction may occur in the transplant because of a blood clot within the distal ureter or bladder, which can be simply relieved by bladder irrigation. Mild hydronephrosis can also be a normal finding in the early transplant kidney as a result of denervation of the collecting system and increased flow thorough the single functioning kidney. It needs to be remembered that the interpretation of any moderate degree of collecting system dilatation should be made only in the presence of an empty bladder, as distension of the bladder alone can be the underlying cause.

In a patient with progressive hydronephrosis and rising creatinine, ureteric obstruction needs to be excluded. Most ureteric obstructions (90%) occur in the distal third of the ureter, reflecting its relatively poor blood supply. The commonest location for a stricture is at the uretero-vesical junction and, where it can be a result of scarring, ischemia, rejection, or surgical technique (Fig. 23).[49] Less commonly, peritransplant collections may compress the ureter, whereas papillary necrosis or fungal balls can obstruct the ureter.[11] It must also be remembered that in the presence of previous or current rejection, sinus edema or fibrosis can prevent the normal hydronephrotic response. Chronic rejection can also mimic a urological complication with rising serum creatinine, and mild pelvicalyceal distension as a result

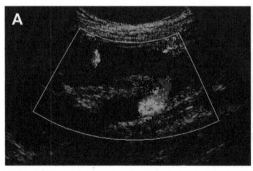
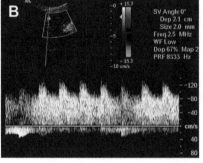

Fig. 21. (A) Two AVFs shown on color-flow imaging with the PRF increased to suppress the Doppler signal from normal vessels. Note the clutter artifact around the larger fistula as a result of tissue vibration. (B) Spectral Doppler trace from the smaller AVF shows a characteristic mixed arterial venous trace.

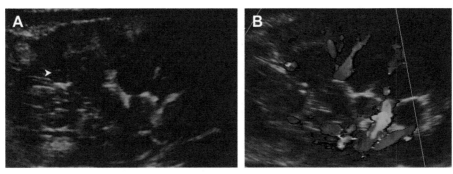

Fig. 22. (*A*) Small cystlike focus seen in a pediatric kidney after intervention for renal calculi. (*B*) Color-flow imaging of this focus shows the typical color reversal sign seen in a pseudoaneurysm.

of cortical thinning. If there is uncertainty regarding the significance of any hydronephrosis seen, measuring the RI within the segmental arteries, might be helpful (ideally should be <0.75), although in the early transplant there are numerous reasons for these to be elevated (see **Table 1**).[13]

Although there remains uncertainty over the diagnosis of obstruction, further imaging with scintigraphy can often be useful in clarifying whether there is normal excretion and drainage of the isotope (eg, mercaptoacetyltriglycine) into the bladder. This can be combined with the administration of a diuretic to enable an assessment of the functional significance of any obstruction present and thereby guide further management.[64] In the case of significant obstruction or where

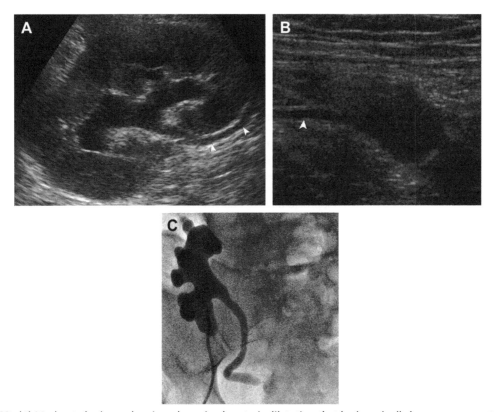

Fig. 23. (*A*) Moderate hydronephrosis and proximal ureteric dilatation that had gradually become apparent over a series of ultrasounds for a poorly functioning graft. Interestingly, the nuclear medicine study was falsely reassuring for normal drainage. (*B*) Zoomed view of the distal ureter (*arrowhead*), which disappears into an area of ill-defined low-reflective (probably fibrotic) tissue. (*C*) Subsequent nephrostomy confirms a tight stricture at the vesicoureteral anastomosis.

there remains uncertainty over the diagnosis in a dilated collecting system, percutaneous puncture of the collecting system should be performed under ultrasound guidance followed by insertion of a nephrostomy if obstruction is confirmed. Following the relief of any ureteric obstruction, the collecting system may remain mildly dilated, making the diagnosis of any further episodes of obstruction challenging. In these situations, a serial change in the degree of dilatation would indicate recurrent obstruction.

CALCULUS DISEASE

The transplant kidney is at increased risk of stone formation, with 1% to 2% developing clinically significant renal caculi.[65] Persisting secondary hyperparathyroidism is seen in a significant number of patients after transplantation and about 15% of transplant patients have persisting hypercalcemia.[66] Therefore, a ureteric calculus should be suspected in the transplant patient with an acute deterioration in renal function. As the kidney is denervated, the patient will not experience typical renal colic. At ultrasonography, the findings are as in the native kidney, with a strongly reflective focus producing acoustic shadowing and twinkling artifact on color Doppler, which may be helpful in confirming small ureteric stones.

NEOPLASMS

Prolonged immunosuppression after renal transplantation carries an increased risk of malignancy of up to 100 times normal for the recipient, with a reported prevalence of 6%.[67] Although this applies to most solid cancers, the commonest seen are skin, cervical, and rectal cancer and lymphomas. Posttransplant lymphoproliferative disorder (PTLD) is seen in about 1% of all transplant patients on long-term immunosuppression and is closely associated with the Epstein-Barr virus. As a result of impaired T-cell function, there is excessive B-cell proliferation, leading to a spectrum of disease from diffuse polyclonal lymphadenopathy to high-grade lymphoma.[68] Extranodal disease is far more common in patients with PTLD, and in renal transplant patients this is often seen in the graft itself. On ultrasonography, PTLD appears as discrete low reflective or mixed reflective masses and tends to have a predilection for the renal hilum. A more diffuse infiltrative pattern can also be seen. Management includes cessation of immunosuppression, antiviral therapy, radiotherapy, and chemotherapy.

Renal cell carcinoma (RCC) has an increased prevalence in the renal transplant population, partly as a result of immunosuppression and partly because of acquired renal cystic disease in the native kidneys. The latter condition is seen in approximately 50% of patients who have been on hemodialysis and although the cysts initially appear simple, they are dysplastic with an approximately 1% risk of malignant change.[69] The cysts can be difficult to see well in often small echogenic kidneys, and if there is any concern then CT should be used for further characterization. De novo RCCs in the allograft are less common and tend to be less aggressive than those seen in the native kidney. Nephron-sparing surgery is the current recommended management, although the use of percutaneous ablative techniques is now being explored (Fig. 24).

RECURRENT RENAL DISEASE

With increasing improvements in length of graft survival, recurrence of the original insult, namely

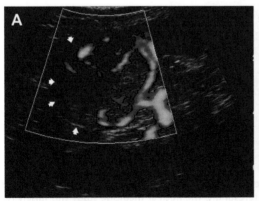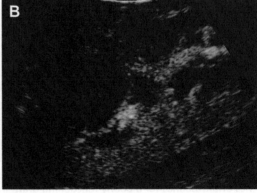

Fig. 24. (A) Ten-year-old transplant that had developed a focal renal mass (arrows) shown to be a low-grade renal cell carcinoma at core biopsy. (B) Contrast-enhanced ultrasound study of same graft following successful radiofrequency ablation of the mass, which completely fails to enhance.

primary glomerulonephritis or secondary renal involvement from a systemic disease may recur. Disease recurrence manifests as proteinuria and decreasing graft function, and is more commonly seen in patients with diabetes, amyloidosis, and cystinosis. Patients with an active vasculitis or oxalosis are at high risk of early recurrent renal damage, which may be viewed as a contraindication to transplantation. There are no specific sonographic findings in recurrent renal disease and its role is confined to excluding the treatable causes discussed previously.

RECENT DEVELOPMENTS IN TRANSPLANT IMAGING

The past 10 years have witnessed a number of new developments in ultrasonography, some of which may have an important role to play in the future assessment of the transplant kidney.

Microbubble Contrast Agents

Microbubble contrast agents are now well established in diagnostic examinations, with the development of low mechanical index (MI) nonlinear imaging modes that exploit particular physical properties of the microbubbles. The suppression of background tissue when using these modes allows areas of tissue enhancement to be clearly identified and, with on- or off-line analysis software, the rate and level of enhancement can now be objectively measured. An additional advantage is that unlike other radiological contrast agents, these agents are not nephrotoxic, being excreted by exhalation and hepatic metabolism.

To date, most work with microbubble contrast agents has focused on characterizing focal liver lesions, with some applications in the native kidney, eg, confirming normal anatomy or distinguishing complex cysts from simple cysts. In the transplant kidney it has been used as a Doppler rescue agent in the standard assessment of transplant blood flow, particularly in the initial postoperative period. The nonlinear imaging modes have also been used to highlight areas of infarction where accessory vessels have failed following surgical anastomosis (**Fig. 25**). However, it is the ability to make a functional assessment of renal blood flow using these agents that is currently attracting most interest.

In the normal transplant kidney following an intravenous injection of microbubble contrast, the renal artery is seen to enhance at about 10 to 20 seconds followed by fairly rapid and marked enhancement of the renal cortex. The medullary pyramids enhance at a much slower rate, remaining relatively echo-poor until late into the

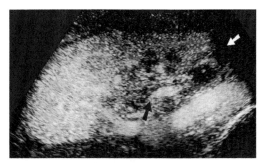

Fig. 25. Contrast-enhanced study of a renal transplant showing normal renal enhancement in the upper pole, reduced perfusion in the interpolar region (*black arrow*) and a small segmental infarct of the lower pole (*white arrow*).

parenchymal phase. Using intermittent bursts of high MI pulses, while scanning over the transplant, destroys the microbubbles present in the image plane so that on returning to a low MI mode the inflow of contrast can be observed again. The quantification software allows regions of interest to be placed over particular areas of the transplant to quantify the rate of contrast inflow, the time to peak enhancement, the area under the enhancement curve, and other parameters (**Fig. 26**). Unlike conventional RI measurements in the interlobar region, this technique has been shown to have very good inter- and intraobserver agreement.[70]

There is now evidence showing that in the early transplant kidney a significant change in the rate of enhancement between the interlobar artery and the renal cortex may allow the distinction to be made between vascular rejection and acute tubular necrosis or nonvascular rejection.[71] There also appears to be a relationship between the estimated glomerular filtration rate and the time delay between enhancement in the renal cortex and that of the medullary pyramids.[72] In the longer term, contrast-enhanced ultrasound (CEUS) of the transplant using the flash replenishment technique to calculate perfusion parameters could prove be much more accurate than renal Doppler RI measurement and serum creatinine in identifying chronic allograft rejection.[73] If confirmed, then this technique will enable early detection of chronic rejection before any rise in creatinine, with the opportunity of therapeutic intervention. The number of studies to date assessing CEUS in the transplant are limited. Further research in this area will be required before this technique becomes accepted as part of the standard imaging protocol for renal allograft imaging. Reassuringly early concerns over possible induced renal interstitial hemorrhage from this technique seem to be unfounded.[74]

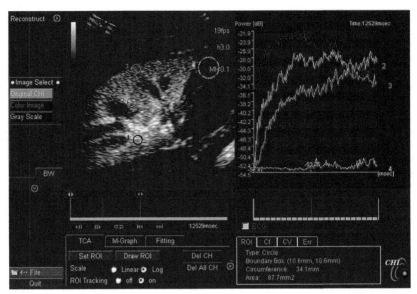

Fig. 26. An example of dynamic enhancement curves taken from various regions of interest in the transplant kidney and one from background tissue, following an injection of a microbubble contrast agent. (*Courtesy of Prof. Thomas Fischer, Berlin.*)

Three-Dimensional Ultrasonography

Three-dimensional ultrasonography of the transplant vasculature may provide useful anatomic information in the assessment of complications, such as large postbiopsy AVF.[75] To date there have been issues with the suppression of flash artifacts in the reconstructed Doppler image, but with the development of novel clutter filter systems, this should become much less of a problem.[76]

Transient Elastography

Transient elastography (TE) is a technique now frequently used in the liver to monitor or detect hepatic fibrosis. A low-frequency vibrating source generates a shear wave within the tissue or organ being assessed and the speed of this wave is measured using a conventional transducer to track tissue displacement. This produces an indirect measurement of tissue stiffness, which can change with certain pathologies. This technique has recently been applied to the transplant kidney to track changes in its tissue stiffness as a result of chronic rejection.[77] Initial results would suggest that TE may be useful in detecting subclinical disease and therefore guiding the nephrologist in when to biopsy.

SUMMARY

Ultrasonography plays a central role in the routine follow-up and complication management of renal transplantation, being the first and often only imaging test required. Its portability enables instant postoperative assessment of blood flow within the graft and evaluation of the vascular anastomoses. Subsequent peritransplant collections can to some extent be characterized and, if required, drained under guidance. Urological complications can be diagnosed and managed almost exclusively with ultrasonography, although CT is now increasingly being used. Color and spectral Doppler can accurately diagnose vascular complications with the addition of microbubble contrast agents where there is uncertainty. By far the main weakness with ultrasonography is its inability to distinguish between the causes of delayed graft function (DGF), usually demonstrating only the nonspecific finding of abnormal internal blood flow and hence not avoiding the need for transplant biopsy. Functional studies with microbubble contrast agents and other recent techniques such as elastography may possibly be able to offer some distinction between the causes of DGF, but further evaluation of these techniques will be required.

REFERENCES

1. Murray JE, Merrill JP, Harrison JH. Kidney transplantation between seven pairs of identical twins. Ann Surg 1958;148:343–59.
2. Starzl TE. Experience in renal transplantation. Philadelphia: WB Saunders; 1964.

3. Khauli RB. Surgical aspects of renal transplantation: new approaches. Urol Clin North Am 1994;21:321–41.

4. Barry JM. Current status of renal transplantation. Patient evaluations and outcomes. Urol Clin North Am 2001;28:677–86.

5. Schuelle P, Lorenz D, Trede M, et al. Impact of renal cadaveric transplantation on survival in end-stage renal failure: evidence for reduced mortality risk compared with haemodialysis during long- term follow-up. J Am Soc Nephrol 1998;9:2135–41.

6. Organ Procurement and Transplantation Network (OPTN. National data, kidney graft/patient survival. OPTN Web site. Available at: http://optn.transplant. hrsa.gov/latestData/viewDataReports.asp. Accessed June 12, 2009.

7. Alexander JW, Zola JC. Expanding the donor pool: use of marginal donors for solid organ transplantation. Clin Transplant 1996;10:1–19.

8. Jimenez C, Lopez MO, Gonzalez E, et al. Ultrasonography in kidney transplantation: values and new developments. Transplant Rev (Orlando) 2009;23:209–13.

9. Carrel A, Guthrie CC. Anastomosis of blood vessels by the patching method and transplantation of the kidney 1906 (classical article). Yale J Biol Med 2001;7:243–7.

10. Cinqualbre J, Kahan BD. René Küss: fifty years of retroperitoneal placement of renal transplants. Transplant Proc 2002;34:3019–25.

11. Akbar SA, Jafri SZH, Amendola MA, et al. Complications of renal transplantation. Radiographics 2005; 25:1335–56.

12. Minnee RC, Bemelman FJ, Laguna Pes PP, et al. Effectiveness of a 5-day external stenting protocol on urological complications after renal transplantation. World J Surg 2009;33:2722–6.

13. Freeman S. The renal transplant. In: Cochlin DL, Dubbins PA, Goldberg BB, et al, editors. Urogenital ultrasound: a text atlas. 2nd edition. Abingdon (UK): Taylor & Francis; 2006. p. 331–56.

14. Cosgrove DO, Chan KE. Renal transplants: what ultrasound can and cannot do. Ultrasound Q 2008; 24:77–87.

15. Rigsby CM, Burns PN, Weltin GG, et al. Doppler signal quantitation in renal allografts: comparison in normal and rejecting transplants, with pathologic correlation. Radiology 1987;162:39–42.

16. Pozniak MA, Kelcz F, Stratta RJ, et al. Extraneous factors affecting resistive index. Invest Radiol 1988;23:899–904.

17. Gao J, Ng A, Shih G, et al. Intrarenal color duplex ultrasonography: a window to vascular complications of renal transplants. J Ultrasound Med 2007; 26:1403–18.

18. Lachance SL, Adamson D, Barry JM. Ultrasonically determined kidney transplant hypertrophy. J Urol 1988;139:497–8.

19. Kok T, Slooff MJ, Thijn CJ, et al. Routine Doppler ultrasound for the detection of clinically unsuspected vascular complications in the early postoperative phase after orthotopic liver transplantation. Transpl Int 1998;11:272.

20. Rifkin MD, Needleman L, Pasto ME, et al. Evaluation of renal transplant rejection by duplex Doppler examination: value of the resistive index. AJR Am J Roentgenol 1987;148:759–62.

21. Genkins S, Sanfilippo F, Carroll B. Duplex Doppler sonography of renal transplants: lack of sensitivity and specificity in establishing pathologic diagnosis. AJR Am J Roentgenol 1989;152:535–9.

22. Choi CS, Lee S, Kim JS, et al. Usefulness of the resistive index for the evaluation of transplanted kidneys. Transplant Proc 1998;30:3074–5.

23. Tublin TE, Bude RO, Platt JF. The resistive index in renal Doppler sonography: where do we stand? AJR Am J Roentgenol 2003;180:885–92.

24. Schwenger V, Keller T, Hofmann N, et al. Color Doppler indices of renal allografts depend on vascular stiffness of the transplant recipients. Am J Transplant 2006;6:2721–4.

25. Akgul A, Sasak G, Basaran C, et al. Relationship of renal resistive index and cardiovascular disease in renal transplant recipients. Transplant Proc 2009; 41:2835–7.

26. Baxter GM, Ireland H, Moss JG, et al. Colour Doppler ultrasound in renal transplant artery stenosis: which Doppler index? Clin Radiol 1995;50:618–22.

27. Merkus JW, Hoitsma AJ, van Asten WN, et al. Doppler spectrum analysis to diagnose rejection during posttransplant acute renal failure. Transplantation 1994;58:570–6.

28. Merkus JW, van Asten WN, Hoitsma AJ, et al. Doppler spectrum analysis in the differential diagnosis of renal transplant dysfunction. Clin Transplant 1996;10:420–8.

29. Daly PJ, Power RE, Healy DA, et al. Delayed graft function: a dilemma in renal transplantation. BJU Int 2005;96:498–501.

30. Lockhart ME, Wells CG, Morgan DE, et al. Reversed diastolic flow in the renal transplant: perioperative implications versus transplants older than 1 month. AJR Am J Roentgenol 2008;190:650–5.

31. Tranquart F, Lebranchu Y, Haillot O, et al. The use of perioperative Doppler ultrasound as a screening test for acute tubular necrosis. Transpl Int 1993;6:14–7.

32. Pirsch JD, Ploeg RJ, Gange S, et al. Determinants of graft survival after renal transplantation. Transplantation 1996;61:1581–5.

33. Cochlin DLL, Wake A, Salaman JR, et al. Ultrasound changes in the transplant kidney. Clin Radiol 1988; 39:373–6.

34. Hilborn MD, Bude RO, Murphy KJ, et al. Renal transplant evaluation with power Doppler sonography. BMJ 1997;70:39–42.

35. Myers BD, Sibley R, Newton L, et al. The long term course of cyclosporine associated chronic nephropathy. Kidney Int 1988;33:590–600.

36. Kumar D. Emerging viruses in transplantation. Curr Opin Infect Dis 2010;23:374–8.

37. Naesens M, Kuypers DR, Sarwal M. Calcineurin inhibitor nephrotoxicity. Clin J Am Soc Nephrol 2009;4:481–508.

38. Kamath NS, John GT, Neelakantan N, et al. Acute graft pyelonephritis following renal transplantation. Transpl Infect Dis 2006;8:140.

39. Lefèvre F, Renoult E, Hubert J, et al. Bladder candidosis after renal transplantation: contribution of ultrasonography. J Radiol 2000;81(4):457–9.

40. Yates PJ, Nicholson ML. The aetiology and pathogenesis of chronic allograft nephropathy. Transpl Immunol 2006;16:148–57.

41. Chapman JR, O'Connell PJ, Nankivell BJ. Chronic renal allograft dysfunction. J Am Soc Nephrol 2005;16:3015–26.

42. Baxter G. Imaging in renal transplantation. Ultrasound Q 2003;19:123–38.

43. Akgul A, Ibis A, Sezer S, et al. Early assessment of renal resistance index and long-term renal function in renal transplant recipients. Ren Fail 2009;31:18–24.

44. Saracino A, Santarsia G, Latorraca A, et al. Early assessment of renal resistance index after kidney transplant can help predict long-term renal function. Nephrol Dial Transplant 2006;21:2916–20.

45. Wilczek HE. Percutaneous needle biopsy of the renal allograft: a clinical safety evaluation of 1129 biopsies. Transplantation 1990;50:790–7.

46. Patel MD, Phillips CJ, Young SW, et al. US-guided renal transplant biopsy: efficacy of a cortical tangential approach. Radiology 2010;256:290–6.

47. Kocak T, Nane I, Ander H, et al. Urologic and surgical complications in 362 consecutive living related donor kidney transplantations. Urol Int 2004;72:252–6.

48. Chung J, Caumartin Y, Warren J, et al. Acute page kidney following renal allograft biopsy: a complication requiring early recognition and treatment. Am J Transplant 2008;8:1323–8.

49. Nargund VH, Cranston D. Urological complications after renal transplantation. Transplant Rev 1996;10:24–33.

50. Singh S, Aoki S, Mitra S, et al. Ascites. An unusual manifestation of urinary leak in a renal allograft recipient. JAMA 1973;226:777–8.

51. Park SB, Kim JK, Cho KS. Complications of renal transplantation: ultrasonographic evaluation. J Ultrasound Med 2007;26:615–33.

52. Król R, Kolonko A, Chudek J, et al. Did volume of lymphocele after kidney transplantation determine the choice of treatment modality? Transplant Proc 2007;39:2740–3.

53. Friedewald SM, Molmenti EP, Friedewald JJ, et al. Vascular and nonvascular complications of renal transplants: sonographic evaluation and correlation with other imaging modalities, surgery, and pathology. J Clin Ultrasound 2005;33:127–9.

54. Kaveggia LP, Perella RR, Grant EG, et al. Duplex Doppler sonography in renal allografts: the significance of reversed flow in diastole. AJR Am J Roentgenol 1990;155:295–8.

55. Rouviere O, Berger P, Beziat C, et al. Acute thrombosis of renal transplant artery: graft salvage by means of intra-arterial fibrinolysis. Transplantation 2002;73:403–9.

56. Jordan ML, Cook GT, Cardella CJ. Ten years of experience with vascular complications in renal transplantation. J Urol 1982;128:689–92.

57. Patel U, Khaw KK, Hughes NC. Doppler ultrasound for detection of renal transplant artery stenosis—threshold peak systolic velocity needs to be higher in a low-risk or surveillance population. Clin Radiol 2003;58:772–7.

58. de Morais RH, Muglia VF, Mamere AE, et al. Duplex Doppler sonography in transplant renal artery stenosis. J Clin Ultrasound 2003;31:135–41.

59. Baxter GM, Morley P, Dall B. Acute renal vein thrombosis in renal allografts: new Doppler ultrasonic findings. Clin Radiol 1991;43:125–7.

60. MacLennan AC, Baxter GM, Harden P, et al. Renal transplant vein occlusion: an early diagnostic sign? Clin Radiol 1995;50:251–3.

61. Brandenburg VM, Frank RD, Riehl J. Color-coded duplex sonography study of arteriovenous fistulae and pseudoaneurysms complicating percutaneous renal allograft biopsy. Clin Nephrol 2002;58:398–404.

62. Harrison KL, Nghiem HV, Coldwell DM, et al. Renal dysfunction due to an arteriovenous fistula in a transplant recipient. J Am Soc Nephrol 1994;5:1300–6.

63. Brown ED, Chen MY, Wolfman NT, et al. Complications of renal transplantation: evaluation with US and radionuclide imaging. Radiographics 2000;20:607–22.

64. Sfakianakis GN, Sfakianaki E, Georgiou M, et al. A renal protocol for all ages and all indications: mercapto-acetyl-triglycine (MAG3) with simultaneous injection of furosemide (MAG3-F0): a 17-year experience. Semin Nucl Med 2009;39:156–73.

65. Cho DK, Zackson DA, Cheigh J, et al. Urinary calculi in renal transplant recipients. Transplantation 1988;45:899–902.

66. de Francisco AM, Riancho JA, Amado JA, et al. Calcium, hyperparathyroidism, and vitamin D metabolism after kidney transplantation. Transplant Proc 1987;19:3721–3.

67. Gallagher MP, Kelly PJ, Jardine M, et al. Long-term cancer risk of immunosuppressive regimens after

kidney transplantation. J Am Soc Nephrol 2010;21: 852–8.

68. Nalesnik MA, Makowka L, Starzl TE, et al. The diagnosis and treatment of posttransplant lymphoproliferative disorders. Curr Probl Surg 1988;25: 371–462.

69. Schwarz A, Vatandaslar S, Merkel S, et al. Renal cell carcinoma in transplant recipients with acquired cystic kidney disease. Clin J Am Soc Nephrol 2007;2:750.

70. Kay DH, Mazonakis M, Geddes C, et al. Ultrasonic microbubble contrast agents and the transplant kidney. Clin Radiol 2009;64:1081–7.

71. Fischer T, Filimonow S, Dieckhöfer J, et al. Improved diagnosis of early kidney allograft dysfunction by ultrasound with echo enhancer: a new method for the diagnosis of renal perfusion. Nephrol Dial Transplant 2006;2:2921–9.

72. Łebkowska U, Janica J, Łebkowski W, et al. Renal parenchyma perfusion spectrum and resistive Index (RI) in ultrasound examinations with contrast medium in the early period after kidney transplantation. Transplant Proc 2009 Oct;41(8):3024–7.

73. Schwenger V, Korosoglou G, Hinkel UP, et al. Real-time contrast enhanced sonography of renal transplant recipients predicts chronic allograft nephropathy. Am J Transplant 2006;6:609–15.

74. Jiménez C, de Gracia R, Aguilera A, et al. In situ kidney insonation with microbubble contrast agents does not cause renal tissue damage in a porcine model. J Ultrasound Med 2008;27:1607–15.

75. Mohaupt MG, Perrig M, Vogt B. 3D ultrasound imaging—a useful non-invasive to detect AV fistulas in transplanted kidneys. Nephrol Dial Transplant 1999;14:940–3.

76. Yoo YM, Sikdar S, Karadayi K, et al. Adaptive clutter rejection for 3D color Doppler imaging: preliminary clinical study. Ultrasound Med Biol 2008;34:1221–31.

77. Arndt R, Schmidt S, Loddenkemper C, et al. Noninvasive evaluation of renal allograft fibrosis by transient elastography—a pilot study. Transpl Int 2010; 3:871–7.

Ultrasound-Guided Therapeutic Urological Interventions

Daniel T. Ginat, MD, MS[a],*, Wael E.A. Saad, MD[b]

KEYWORDS

- Ultrasound • Renal • Cyst • Aspiration • Sclerosis
- Nephrostomy • Suprapubic cystostomy

Interventional uroradiology is a well-established discipline that offers minimally invasive treatment options for a wide spectrum of urinary system conditions.[1,2] Many interventional uroradiology procedures are amenable to ultrasound guidance, either alone or in combination with other modalities, such as fluoroscopy and computed tomography (CT). The use of ultrasound guidance is particularly desirable because of its low cost, accurate real-time target visualization, and lack of ionizing radiation. Furthermore, many procedures are more safely and rapidly performed with ultrasound guidance.[3] In this article, indications, techniques, and outcomes of ultrasound-guided nephrostomy, cyst aspiration, sclerotherapy, and suprapubic catheterization are reviewed and illustrated.

NEPHROSTOMY

Ultrasound-guided percutaneous nephrostomy (PCN) is a minimally invasive procedure in which the pelvicalyceal system is accessed to provide external urinary drainage or a route for minimally invasive procedures. Indications for PCN include urinary diversion for urinary tract obstruction, nephrolithiasis, urinary tract infections, urinary fistulas, hemorrhagic cystitis, and ureteral injuries,

as well as to provide a percutaneous portal for more advanced interventions, including stone extraction, lithotripsy, and ureteroscopy.[3–6] Infected urinary tract obstruction is an urgent indication for PCN. The main contraindication to PCN is severe coagulopathy.[7]

Preparation for PCN includes reviewing available imaging studies to evaluate the location, anatomy, and orientation of the target kidney. In the presence of renal dysfunction, a noncontrast CT scan is still valuable. This type of study can identify and delineate the extent of subcapsular hematoma, uncontained retroperitoneal hemorrhage, and gross hematuria in the collecting system, as manifested by high-attenuation material. Ideally, patients should be made to fast for 6 to 8 hours before the procedure and intravenous access should be obtained. Most patients tolerate PCN with moderate conscious sedation and local anesthesia; general anesthesia is usually not required. Patients are typically positioned prone or oblique prone, and the target kidney is imaged using ultrasound to assess its location and anatomy again. Ultrasound-guided PCN can be successfully performed in patients with nondilated pelvicalyceal systems after diuretic administration, which provides transient distension.[8] The skin at the access site is prepared and draped following

The authors have no conflicts of interest to disclose.

[a] Department of Imaging Sciences, University of Rochester Medical Center, 601 Elmwood Avenue, Box 648, Rochester, NY 14642, USA

[b] Department of Radiology, University of Virginia Health System, 1215 Lee Street, PO Box 800170, Charlottesville, VA 22908, USA

* Corresponding author.

E-mail address: daniel_ginat@urmc.rochester.edu

Ultrasound Clin 5 (2010) 401–408

doi:10.1016/j.cult.2010.04.001

surgical standards. After infiltrating the region of interest with local anesthetic, a small skin incision is made using a scalpel.

Needle access for PCN can be achieved entirely by ultrasound guidance (**Fig. 1**), which is of comparable efficacy to fluoroscopic guidance and may be associated with fewer complications.[9,10] Attempting to perform PCN solely by ultrasound guidance with minimal fluoroscopy is especially desirable in pregnant patients. However, fluoroscopy is the guidance modality of choice for percutaneous nephrolithotripsy.

A posterior calyx located below the level of the 11th rib should be selected for access to the collecting system.[11] An 18- to 22-gauge access needle is oriented in a 20° to 30° posterolateral oblique approach along the avascular plane of Brödel and passed directly into the target calyx under real-time ultrasound guidance, using a single-stick technique.[11] Large-caliber needles are recommended for definitive access because they are more likely to maintain a straight path toward the target calyx during ultrasound-guided insertion.[12] Furthermore, 18- to 19-gauge needles accept the 0.035-in wires that are used for dilators and nephrostomy tubes. Alternatively, direct access to the collecting system can be obtained using a trocar system technique under ultrasound

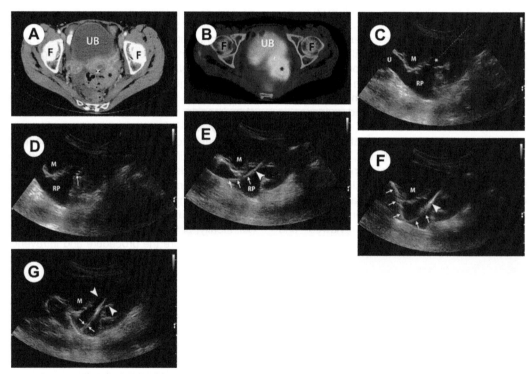

Fig. 1. Ultrasound-guided definitive needle access for PCN. (*A, B*) Axial contrast-enhanced CT image (*A*) and a positron emission tomography-CT image (*B*) at the level of the femoral heads (F) of a patient with left pelvic mass (*asterisk*) obstructing the left ureter in its distal course as it approaches the urinary bladder (UB). The malignant mass takes up radiotracer (*asterisk*). (*C*) Gray-scale ultrasound image of the left kidney with the operator centered at the lower pole calyx (*asterisk*). A dashed line is drawn to show the needle trajectory that is planned. Above the target calyx (*asterisk*) lies the mid to lower pole calyx (M). The upper pole calyx (U) is observed continuous with the renal pelvis (RP) that lies deep to the mid and lower calyces. (*D*) Gray-scale ultrasound image of the left kidney of the same patient. The operator has passed an 18-gauge needle (*arrow* at needle tip) directly into the lower pole calyx. (M indicates mid to lower pole calyx, RP indicates renal pelvis). (*E, F*) Gray-scale ultrasound image of the left kidney of the same patient. The operator has passed a 0.035-in guidewire (*arrows*) through the 18-gauge needle (*arrowhead* at needle tip) that is in the lower pole calyx. At this point of the procedure, fluoroscopy is used as the image-guidance modality. (*G*) Gray-scale ultrasound image of the left kidney of the same patient. This is an image obtained after the 8F nephrostomy drain (between *arrows*) has been placed through the lower pole calyx (between *arrowheads*) and into the RP.

visualization.[13] The following steps comprise the remainder of the procedure:

- Advancement of a metal wire through the access needle with sufficient purchase. A safety wire is sometimes added for complicated procedures, whereby the tip is positioned in the distal ureter or urinary bladder. Double-wire access is gained by passing a 6F to 7F sheath over the original wire down the ureter and inserting the second wire parallel to the first wire within the sheath, which can then be removed.
- Removal of the needle over the guidewire.
- Insertion of a fascial dilator that is 2 gauges wider than the nephrostomy tube. Balloon angioplasty of the tract can be performed as well.
- Removal of dilator/balloon over guidewire.
- Insertion of the nephrostomy tube with the distal end positioned and looped within the renal pelvis.
- The nephrostomy tube is secured to the skin with sutures and left to gravity bag drainage.
- Immediate postprocedure fluoroscopy or ultrasound should be performed to document appropriate positioning of the nephrostomy tube within the renal pelvis. If necessary, repositioning of the catheter is performed under fluoroscopy.

Two-step needle access using ultrasound-guided access of the renal pelvis followed by definitive fluoroscopy-guided needle access is an alternative technique that is not commonly implemented. This technique is reserved for situations in which there is not much or no calyceal dilation and when intravenous contrasts delineating the renal collecting system cannot be administered. Ultrasound is used to guide a 21- to 22-gauge needle into the renal pelvis. Contrast is then injected into the renal collecting system. Air can also be injected to delineate the posterior calyces with the patient prone. Definitive needle access into the inferior renal calyces is then achieved under fluoroscopy. The advantage of ultrasound localization and access is that it is in real time and does not rely on landmarks. Indeed, the kidney can change in position with moderate sedation, leading to inaccurate access on the basis of fluoroscopic landmarks based on preprocedural CT images.

The technical success rate for ultrasound-guided PCN performed by interventional radiologists is about 98%.[14,15] Similarly, ultrasound-guided percutaneous nephrolithotomy has a stone-free success rate of 96.5%. Major

complications occur in 0% to 5.6% of patients after PCN, which include hemorrhage requiring transfusion and sepsis.[15–17]

Major hemorrhage occurs in less than 4% of the cases and may be associated with pseudoaneurysm formation. This condition requires additional investigation and possible intervention, such as angiography and possible embolization. Septic shock occurs in less than 4% of patients but is the most severe complication of PCN.[18,19] The overall mortality rate related to PCN is estimated at 0.04%.[11]

Minor complications occur in up to 28% of the cases,[20] which include catheter displacement or malposition, pelvic perforation, ileus, urinary tract infection, catheter obstruction by debris, urinary leakage, skin inflammation insertion site, and pleural effusion. Each of these complications typically occurs in 1% to 5% of the cases.[21] Percutaneous nephrolithotomy has an early complication rate of more than 50%, mainly attributable to transient fever (28%) and urinary tract infection (3.5%).[16]

CT angiography is the most suitable initial modality for evaluating complications related to PCN, particularly in emergent cases.[22,23] The technique is effective for diagnosing postprocedure hemorrhage and can often localize the site of bleeding. Doppler ultrasound, conventional angiography, and CT angiography are all appropriate modalities for identifying arteriovenous fistulas. However, the advantage of conventional arteriography is that concomitant treatment by transcatheter embolization can be performed.[24]

RENAL CYST ASPIRATION AND SCLEROTHERAPY

Simple renal cysts are common in the general population, with an overall prevalence of 11.9% to 17.2% on ultrasound examination.[25–27] With age, simple renal cysts increase in prevalence, size, and number, affecting 22.1% to 36.1% of individuals older than 70 years.[25,27,28] Although most simple renal cysts are incidental findings, these lesions occasionally produce symptoms including flank pain, hypertension, hematuria, and hydronephrosis.[29–35] Symptomatic renal cysts are amenable to percutaneous aspiration and sclerotherapy if the imaging features satisfy the Bosniak criteria for benignity.[36] Patients with polycystic kidney disease may also benefit from the procedure.[29] Preprocedural imaging is also useful for excluding other possible causes for the symptoms.

Cyst aspiration can be performed alone or in combination with sclerotherapy. It has been recommended that a trial of aspiration be performed, followed by sclerosis, if there is recurrence. However, the recurrence rate for aspiration alone is up to 80%.[37] Consequently, sclerotherapy is routinely performed in conjunction with aspiration during the same session. The first and most widely used sclerosing agent for treating simple renal cysts is 95% ethanol.[38] The authors have had successful results with doxycycline (500 mg) combined with 1% lidocaine (5 mL). Numerous other agents have been applied toward renal cyst treatment, with varying degrees of success (Table 1). Alternatively, continuous negative pressure has been described.[39] These techniques can be performed under local anesthesia, with or without conscious sedation. The following are the general procedural steps for cyst aspiration and sclerotherapy:

- Localization of the cyst under ultrasound, usually with the patient positioned on the side or supine.
- Introduction of a multi-sidehole pigtail catheter (typically 8F) into the cyst cavity using the trocar method under ultrasound guidance.
- Withdrawing the maximum cyst fluid. Repositioning the patient may optimize the yield.
- The amount of fluid removed should be recorded and samples should be sent for microbial and cytologic analysis.
- Up to 50% of diluted contrast material should be injected into the cyst to rule out communication with the pelvicalyceal system or leakage.

- If there is indeed a communication or leakage, the procedure is discontinued. Otherwise, the contrast material is aspirated and a small amount (5 mL) of lidocaine may be injected for pain relief, if necessary.
- Injection of sclerosing agent with 10% to 40% of the initial cyst volume, but usually no more than 100 to 200 mL.
- Aspiration of sclerosing agent after 5 minutes to 4 hours, depending on the particular agent used.
- Repeat sclerosant injections can be performed.

In general, the various techniques for simple renal cyst aspiration and sclerotherapy are safe and effective. Single-session ethanol sclerotherapy eliminates hydronephrosis in 83.3% of cases, resolves hypertension in 87.5% of cases, and mitigates pain in 90% of cases.[32] A second intervention is necessary in 2% of cases because of recurrence.[32] Success rates may be improved by repeated sessions of ethanol sclerotherapy,[40] higher concentrations of ethanol,[41] longer dwell times of up to 4 hours,[42] and the use of continuous negative pressure.[39] Satisfactory results with dwell times as brief as 5 minutes can be achieved with agents such as acetic acid. Other agents, such as OK-432, cause less pain than ethanol during the procedure.[43] Regardless of the sclerosant used, cyst size also determines success, as larger cysts are more likely to recur.[44]

Most studies do not report any major complications related to simple renal cyst aspiration and sclerotherapy. In rare instances, nephrocutaneous

Table 1
Assortment of sclerosing agents for simple renal cyst treatment

Sclerosant	Comments
95% ethanol	Most commonly used agent
99% ethanol	Simple, fast, safe, effective, inexpensive
STDS	Less painful than ethanol
Povidone-iodine	High rate of recurrence
NBCA and iodized oil	Simple, safe, effective, well tolerated
OK-432	Simpler, safer, and more effective than multiple session 99% ethanol sclerotherapy
50% acetic acid	Effective and safe; 5 min dwell time
EOI mixture	Possibly safe, effective, well tolerated
3% polidocanol (Aethoxysklerol)	Less expensive than ethanol and has no side effects, but tends to lead to septic complications
Continuous negative pressure	More efficient than single-session alcohol sclerotherapy for giant cysts

Abbreviations: EOI, ethanolamine oleate-iopamidol; NBCA, *N*-butyl cyanoacrylate; STDS, sodium tetradecyl sulfate.

fistulas and urinary tract infections have occurred in association with cyst aspiration and sclerotherapy.[29] A sensation of drunkenness and fever has been described after ethanol sclerotherapy.[45] Follow-up imaging for evaluation of the residual cyst size and most complications related to the procedure is generally performed by CT.

CYSTORETROPERITONEAL SHUNTING

Ultrasound-guided percutaneous cystoretroperitoneal shunting is a recently described treatment for simple renal cysts. The technique consists of decompressing the cyst contents into the retroperitoneal space on a long-term basis, similar to laparoscopic cyst decortication or marsupialization. Essentially, the same patient preparation as for ultrasound-guided percutaneous renal cyst aspiration is necessary for this technique. As described by Canguven and colleagues,[46] cystoretroperitoneal shunting is performed by the following steps:

- A ring drainage ring catheter with multiple sideholes is inserted into the cyst by a small flank puncture.
- The tip of the drainage catheter is positioned against the opposite cyst wall.
- A maximum amount of cyst fluid is aspirated and sent for laboratory analysis.
- The drainage catheter is sutured at 2 subcutaneous sites.
- The drainage catheter is usually removed after 3 months.
- Sclerotherapy can be performed in conjunction with the initial catheter insertion or along with repeat cyst aspiration, if there is recurrence.

Preliminary results indicate a 100% technical success rate for this procedure.[46] Pain relief and blood pressure control are achieved in 80.5% and 46.1% of cases, respectively, after catheter removal. However, 36.2% of cysts recur by 16 months. Inadvertent migration of the catheter outside the cyst cavity and consequent recurrence was found in less than 3% of cases. Further study of this technique and the use of biodegradable catheters are warranted.

SUPRAPUBIC CYSTOSTOMY

Indications for percutaneous suprapubic cystostomy include bladder outlet obstruction, traumatic avulsion of the urinary bladder from its neck or, in cases of posttraumatic bladder leakage, to provide a route for removing urinary bladder stones (cystolithotomy), fulgurating superficial premalignant lesions in the urinary bladder, antegrade cannulation of the urethra to guide retrograde cannulation of the urinary bladder, and bladder aspiration for fever workup. An advantage of suprapubic catheters over transurethral catheterization is that suprapubic catheters can be clamped to test for the patient's ability to void without losing access or subjecting the patient to another retrograde Foley catheter placement. A relative contraindication to suprapubic cystostomy is uncorrected coagulopathy, and an absolute contraindication is status after total cystectomy. Preprocedural imaging evaluation consists of confirming the location of the bladder and availability of a percutaneous window to the urinary bladder. In particular, the skin access site is selected by triangulating the position of the urinary bladder, preferably through the midline at the linea alba, which is the least vascular plane.

Ultrasound-guided access can be obtained using multiarray 4- to 5-MHz transducer with guide bracket and a sterile transducer cover. After standard surgical preparation and draping, the followings steps are performed (**Fig. 2**):

- A vertical skin incision is made using a scalpel to facilitate trocar or needle insertion.
- Via freehand ultrasound guidance, a needle (usually 18-gauge) connected to a 20-mL syringe containing contrast material is inserted without a stylet.
- Once the needle traverses the subcutaneous tissues, suction is applied as the needle is advanced. The use of connector tubing allows the operator to have flexibility while manipulating the needle freehand.
- Entry of the needle tip into the urinary bladder can be visualized with real-time ultrasound and is confirmed by an abrupt return of urine into the syringe.
- A urine sample can be obtained and sent for analysis, if necessary.
- Subsequently, radiographic contrast is injected under fluoroscopy to confirm adequate placement of the needle into the urinary bladder.
- If the Seldinger technique is implemented, a 0.035-in or 0.038-in wire is introduced through the needle, which is then exchanged over an 8F to 12F self-retaining pigtail drainage catheter.
- Fascial dilators are sized according to the final size of the percutaneous drain.
- The pigtail is then inserted over the guidewire, which is then removed.

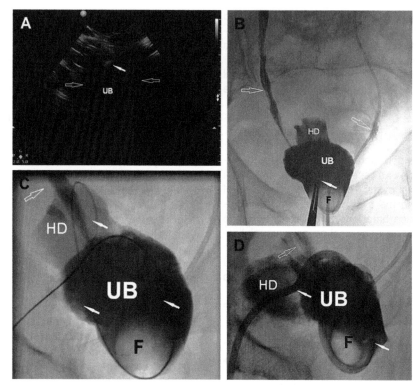

Fig. 2. (*A*) Transverse gray-scale ultrasound image of urinary bladder (UB, between *hollow arrows*) being filled retrograde by Foley catheter with diluted contrast. The 18-gauge needle tip (*solid arrow*) is being inserted into the urinary bladder. (*B*) Fluoroscopic image with contrast in the urinary bladder. A clamp is placed holding the needle (*solid arrow*). Contrast is seen filling the urinary bladder (UB), encircling the balloon of the Foley catheter (F), filling a Hutch diverticulum (HD), and refluxing bilaterally up the stented ureters (*hollow arrows*). (*C*) Oblique fluoroscopic image with a 0.035-in wire coiled (*solid arrows*) in the urinary bladder. Again seen is contrast filling the urinary bladder (UB), encircling the balloon of the Foley catheter (F), filling a Hutch diverticulum (HD), and refluxing up the stented right ureter (*hollow arrow*). (*D*) Oblique fluoroscopic image with a 0.035-in wire coiled (*solid arrows*) in the urinary bladder. Again seen is contrast filling the urinary bladder (UB), encircling the balloon of the Foley catheter (F), filling a Hutch diverticulum (HD), and refluxing up the stented right ureter (*hollow arrow*).

- Once the distal end is positioned in the urinary bladder, the catheter is coped, secured to the skin with sutures, and left to gravity bag drainage.
- Immediate postdrainage imaging is usually performed with fluoroscopy to confirm that the pigtail suprapubic catheter is appropriately positioned within the urinary bladder and that it is well formed.

Technical success is achieved in more than 90% of cases, even in emergent situations.[47] Technical failures are more common with thick trabeculated bladder wall, where the operator has been able to access the bladder with the needle but has found difficulty passing a drain. This difficulty can be mitigated with the use of a peel-away sheath. Ultrasound-guided suprapubic cystostomy is generally a safe procedure.

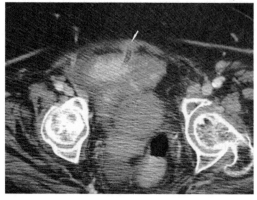

Fig. 3. Axial CT image demonstrates the suprapubic catheter within the small bowel (*arrow*).

Complications among patients with spinal cord injury include gross hematuria in 20%, febrile urinary tract infections in 15%, urosepsis in 10%, pyelonephritis in 4%, and leakage around the suprapubic tube insertion site in 26%.[48] Revision of the suprapubic tube is required in 13% of such cases.[48] With ultrasound guidance, bowel perforation (**Fig. 3**) and other manifestations of suprapubic catheter malpositions are very rare.

SUMMARY

Ultrasound increases the speed, safety, and accuracy of percutaneous urological interventions without imparting radiation dose. Ultrasound-guided PCN, renal cyst aspiration and sclerotherapy, and suprapubic cystostomy are generally regarded as effective, minimally invasive options for managing various diseases of the urinary tract. Ongoing developments of these techniques will continue to expand the breadth of applications and success of ultrasound-guided urological interventions.

REFERENCES

1. Kang P, Paspulati R. Ultrasound-guided genitourinary interventions. Ultrasound Clin 2007;2:115–20.
2. Dyer RB, Assimos DG, Regan JD. Update on interventional uroradiology. Urol Clin North Am 1997;24: 623–52.
3. Porcaro W, Tibbles CD. Procedural applications of ultrasound. Emerg Med Clin North Am 2004;22: 797–815.
4. Dyer RB, Regan JD, Kavanagh PV, et al. Percutaneous nephrostomy with extensions of the technique: step by step. Radiographics 2002; 22:503–25.
5. Hausegger KA, Portugaller HR. Percutaneous nephrostomy and antegrade ureteral stenting: technique—indications—complications. Eur Radiol 2006; 16:2016–30.
6. Avritscher R, Madoff DC, Ramirez PT, et al. Fistulas of the lower urinary tract: percutaneous approaches for the management of a difficult clinical entity. Radiographics 2004;24:S217–36.
7. Stables DP, Ginsberg NJ, Johnson ML. Percutaneous nephrostomy: a series and review of the literature. AJR Am J Roentgenol 1978;130:75–82.
8. Gupta S, Gulati M, Suri S. Ultrasound-guided percutaneous nephrostomy in non-dilated pelvicalyceal system. J Clin Ultrasound 1998;26:177–9.
9. Basiri A, Ziaee AM, Kianian HR, et al. Ultrasonographic versus fluoroscopic access for percutaneous nephrolithotomy: a randomized clinical trial. J Endourol 2008;22:281–4.
10. Hosseini MM, Hassanpour A, Farzan R, et al. Ultrasonography-guided percutaneous nephrolithotomy. J Endourol 2009;23:603–7.
11. Zagoria RJ, Dyer RB. Do's and don't's of percutaneous nephrostomy. Acad Radiol 1999;6:370–7.
12. Saad WE, Moorthy M, Ginat D. Percutaneous nephrostomy: native and transplanted kidneys. Tech Vasc Interv Radiol 2009;12:172–92.
13. Newhouse JH, Pfister RC. Percutaneous catheterization of the kidney and perinephric space: trocar technique. Urol Radiol 1981;2:157–64.
14. Martino P. Ultrasound-guided percutaneous nephrostomy. Arch Ital Urol Androl 2000;72:324–7.
15. Montanari E, Serrago M, Esposito N, et al. Ultrasound-fluoroscopy guided access to the intrarenal excretory system. Ann Urol (Paris) 1999;33:168–81.
16. Skolarikos A, Alivizatos G, Papatsoris A, et al. Ultrasound-guided percutaneous nephrostomy performed by urologists: 10-year experience. Urology 2006;68:495–9.
17. Gupta S, Gulati M, Uday Shankar K, et al. Percutaneous nephrostomy with real-time sonographic guidance. Acta Radiol 1997;38:454–7.
18. Patel U, Hussain FF. Percutaneous nephrostomy of nondilated renal collecting systems with fluoroscopic guidance: technique and results. Radiology 2004;233:226–33.
19. Lewis S, Patel U. Major complications after percutaneous nephrostomy—lessons from a department audit. Clin Radiol 2004;59:171–9.
20. Sood G, Sood A, Jindal A, et al. Ultrasound guided percutaneous nephrostomy for obstructive uropathy in benign and malignant diseases. Int Braz J Urol 2006;32:281–6.
21. Lee WJ, Patel U, Patel S, et al. Emergency percutaneous nephrostomy: results and complications. J Vasc Interv Radiol 1994;5:135–9.
22. Harris RD, Walther PC. Renal arterial injury associated with percutaneous nephrostomy. Urology 1984;23:215–7.
23. Sadick M, Röhrl B, Schnülle P, et al. Multislice CT-angiography in percutaneous postinterventional hematuria and kidney bleeding: influence of diagnostic outcome on therapeutic patient management. Preliminary results. Arch Med Res 2007;38: 126–32.
24. Vignali C, Lonzi S, Bargellini I, et al. Vascular injuries after percutaneous renal procedures: treatment by transcatheter embolization. Eur Radiol 2004;14:723–9.
25. Terada N, Ichioka K, Matsuta Y, et al. The natural history of simple renal cysts. J Urol 2002;167:21–3.
26. Caglioti A, Esposito C, Fuiano G, et al. Prevalence of symptoms in patients with simple renal cysts. BMJ 1993;306:430–1.
27. Terada N, Arai Y, Kinukawa N, et al. The 10-year natural history of simple renal cysts. Urology 2008; 71:7–11.

28. Ravine D, Gibson RN, Donlan J, et al. An ultrasound renal cyst prevalence survey: specificity data for inherited renal cystic diseases. Am J Kidney Dis 1993;22:803–7.

29. Singh I, Mehrotra G. Selective ablation of symptomatic dominant renal cysts using 99% ethanol in adult polycystic kidney disease. Urology 2006;68:482–7.

30. Mohsen T, Gomha MA. Treatment of symptomatic simple renal cysts by percutaneous aspiration and ethanol sclerotherapy. BJU Int 2005;96:1369–72.

31. Bennett WM, Elzinga L, Golper TA, et al. Reduction of cyst volume for symptomatic management of autosomal dominant polycystic kidney disease. J Urol 1987;137:620–2.

32. Akinci D, Akhan O, Ozmen M, et al. Long-term results of single-session percutaneous drainage and ethanol sclerotherapy in simple renal cysts. Eur J Radiol 2005;54:298–302.

33. Hoard TD, O'Brien DP 3rd. Simple renal cyst and high renin hypertension cured by cyst decompression. J Urol 1976;115:326–7.

34. Churchill D, Kimoff R, Pinsky M, et al. Solitary intrarenal cyst: correctable cause of hypertension. Urology 1975;6:485–8.

35. Akinci D, Gumus B, Ozkan OS, et al. Single-session percutaneous ethanol sclerotherapy in simple renal cysts in children: long-term follow-up. Pediatr Radiol 2005;35:155–8.

36. Bosniak MA. The current radiological approach to renal cysts. Radiology 1986;158:1–10.

37. Hanna RM, Dahniya MH. Aspiration and sclerotherapy of symptomatic simple renal cysts: value of two injections of sclerosing agents. AJR Am J Roentgenol 1996;167:781–3.

38. Bean WJ. Renal cysts: treatment with alcohol. Radiology 1981;138:329–31.

39. Zerem E, Imamović G, Omerović S. Symptomatic simple renal cyst: comparison of continuous negative-pressure catheter drainage and single-session alcohol sclerotherapy. AJR Am J Roentgenol 2008; 190:1193–7.

40. Chung BH, Kim JH, Hong CH, et al. Comparison of single and multiple sessions of percutaneous sclerotherapy for simple renal cyst. BJU Int 2000;85: 626–7.

41. Gasparini D, Sponza M, Valotto C, et al. Renal cysts: can percutaneous ethanol injections be considered an alternative to surgery? Urol Int 2003;71:197–200.

42. Lin YH, Pan HB, Liang HL, et al. Single-session alcohol-retention sclerotherapy for simple renal cysts: comparison of 2- and 4-hr retention techniques. AJR Am J Roentgenol 2005;185:860–6.

43. Demir E, Alan C, Kilciler M, et al. Comparison of ethanol and sodium tetradecyl sulfate in the sclerotherapy of renal cyst. J Endourol 2007;21: 903–5.

44. El-Diasty TA, Shokeir AA, Tawfeek HA, et al. Ethanol sclerotherapy for symptomatic simple renal cysts. J Endourol 1995;9:273–6.

45. Cho DS, Ahn HS, Kim SI, et al. Sclerotherapy of renal cysts using acetic acid: a comparison with ethanol sclerotherapy. Br J Radiol 2008;81:946–9.

46. Canguven O, Goktas C, Yencilek F, et al. A new technique for simple renal cyst: cystoretroperitoneal shunt. Adv Urol 2009:906013.

47. Peate I. Patient management following suprapubic catheterization. Br J Nurs 1997;6:555–62.

48. Katsumi HK, Kalisvaart JF, Ronningen LD, et al. Urethral versus suprapubic catheter: choosing the best bladder management for male spinal cord injury patients with indwelling catheters. Spinal Cord 2010;48:325–9.

Ultrasonography for Fetal Genitourinary Abnormalities: The Essentials

Alka S. Karnik, MD*, Anjumara Bora, DMRE, DNB

KEYWORDS

- Antenatal ultrasound • Oligohydramnios • Pelvicaliectasis
- Vesicoureteric reflux • Cystic dysplasia • Renal masses
- Adrenal masses • Ambiguous genitalia

Embryologically the urogenital system develops from a common mesodermal ridge; however, functionally and structurally there are two distinct systems, the urinary system and the genital system. Ultrasonography is an excellent modality for detection and characterization of urinary tract abnormalities, which occur in 3% to 4% of the population and form 30% of the abnormalities detected on a routine antenatal ultrasonography.[1] Lethal urinary tract abnormalities account for 10% of pregnancy terminations. Early antenatal detection and serial follow-up help in obstetric and neonatal management.[2] The typical morphology of various abnormalities helps in accurate prenatal diagnosis and in selected cases MR imaging gives valuable information.[3] Genital evaluation and determination of gender is important in cases of several morphologic anomalies. In ambiguous genitalia, there is often inability to assign fetal gender in a second- or third-trimester sonographic examination.

URINARY TRACT—NORMAL SONOGRAPHIC ANATOMY

Fetal kidneys can be visualized in the first trimester. On a combined transabdominal/transvaginal scan at 12 to 13 weeks, kidneys are seen in 99% of cases as oval structures in the paravertebral region and appear relatively hyperechoic compared with the liver and spleen (Fig. 1A). In second trimester, kidneys are well seen on transabdominal sonography as iso/hypoechoic oval structures with an echogenic renal sinus and echogenic borders due to perinephric fat (see Fig. 1B). Corticomedullary distinction becomes apparent in the second trimester and is well marked in third-trimester scans (see Fig. 1C). A central lucency due to presence of fluid in the renal pelvis is often seen. Under normal conditions, the ureters are not visible.[4–6] The renal length in millimeters is equal to gestational age in weeks from 24 weeks and onwards. Renal growth can also be normally evaluated by measuring length and comparing it to available normograms.[5]

The urinary bladder is visualized on a transabdominal examination at 12 to 13 weeks of gestation. The bladder volume is normally 1 mL at 20 weeks and increases to 36 mL at 41 weeks, with bladder emptying observed at approximately every 25 minutes.[4,5] On a color Doppler examination, two umbilical arteries are seen, one on each side of the urinary bladder (Fig. 2).

Amniotic fluid is an important indicator of fetal renal and placental function. After 16 weeks, fetal urine production is the major source of amniotic fluid.[7] Oligohydramnios is often the first sign of a renal anomaly when there is significantly compromised function. When there is a detected renal abnormality, the presence of normal amniotic fluid indicates good prognosis.

Radiology, Department of Ultrasound, Dr Balabhai Nanavati Hospital and Research Center, Vileparle West, Mumbai 400057, Maharashtra, India
* Corresponding author.
E-mail address: drakarnik@rediffmail.com

Ultrasound Clin 5 (2010) 409–425
doi:10.1016/j.cult.2010.08.003
1556-858X/10/$ — see front matter © 2010 Published by Elsevier Inc.

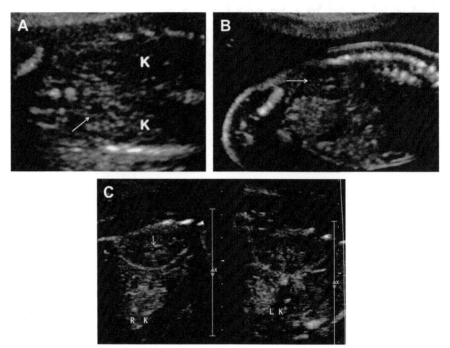

Fig. 1. (*A*) At 14 weeks' gestation, coronal image shows fetal kidneys (K) as oval structures in the paravertebral region relatively hyperechoic as compared with the liver (*arrow*). (*B*) In the second trimester, the kidneys are iso/hypoechoic with an echogenic renal sinus and echogenic border due to perinephric fat (*arrow*). Corticomedullary differentiation is seen. (*C*) Third-trimester sagittal image shows good renal corticomedullary differentiation. A central lucency due to fluid in the renal pelvis is often seen (*arrow*). LK, left kidney; RK, right kidney.

ULTRASONOGRAPHY DIAGNOSIS OF URINARY TRACT ABNORMALITIES—WHAT TO LOOK FOR

Box 1 details the assessment protocol for the diagnosis of urinary tract abnormalities.

Empty Renal Fossa

Failure of ureteric bud to induce metanephric blastema leads to renal agenesis. On careful

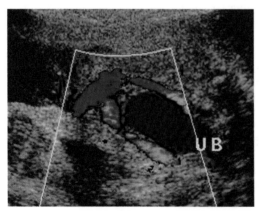

Fig. 2. Axial color Doppler image demonstrates the normal urinary bladder (UB) flanked by umbilical arteries.

Box 1
Ultrasonography diagnosis of urinary tract abnormalities—What to look for

1. Assessment of amniotic fluid volume
2. Localization and characterization of urinary tract abnormalities

   Bladder seen earlier than the kidneys

   - Presence
   - Appearance and size

   Kidneys sagittal/transverse

   - Presence
   - Number
   - Position
   - Size
   - Appearance (echogenicity and cysts)
   - Unilateral or bilateral

   Collecting system

   - Dilatation
   - Level of obstruction
   - Cause of obstruction
   - Unilateral or bilateral

3. Fetal gender
4. Two-vessel umbilical cord often seen with renal anomalies
5. Search for associated abnormalities

assessment of the renal fossa, absence of renal tissue is first seen on an axial view and confirmed on a longitudinal view. The adrenal glands may fill the renal fossa and be mistaken for dysplastic kidneys. Typically, lying down adrenals with long axis parallel to the spine are often noted.[8] These are large and globular and the normal Y shape is not seen.[9,10] Renal absence may be unilateral or bilateral. Unilateral agenesis accounts for 54% of cases of empty renal fossa, ectopic pelvic kidney for 37%, fusion abnormalities (eg, horseshoe kidney) for 5%, and cross-fused ectopia for 4%.

Bilateral Renal Agenesis (Potter syndrome)

Bilateral renal agenesis is a lethal abnormality. The diagnosis is based initially on anhydramnios at 15 weeks' gestation, nonvisualization of renal structures bilaterally,[9] and a persistently empty urinary bladder. Rarely there may be a small amount of fluid due to retrograde filling of the bladder. On color Doppler ultrasonography, the renal arteries are not visualized (**Fig. 3**).[11] In difficult cases, MR imaging helps confirm renal absence.[3] Anhydramnios leads to other abnormalities, including pulmonary hypoplasia with an altered chest/cardiac ratio, typical Potter facies, and musculoskeletal abnormalities (club feet and joint contractures). Associated congenital heart disease anomalies occur in 14% of cases. Renal agenesis may also be part of the VACTERL association: *v*ertebral, *a*norectal, and *c*ardiac anomalies; *t*rachea-esophageal fistula; and *r*enal and *l*imb anomalies. A two-vessel umbilical cord is often seen.

Unilateral Renal Agenesis

In unilateral renal agenesis, the amount of liquor is normal and there is a single empty renal fossa, the left (57%) more common than right.[12] There is compensatory hypertrophy of the single kidney with size greater than 95th percentile, seen as early as 22 weeks (**Fig. 4**).[13] Color Doppler confirms an absent renal artery, best visualized on the coronal aorta view. The adrenal glands or on the left side, the colon, in the empty renal fossa may mimic a kidney.[10]

Abnormal Position

The amount of liquor is normal with an empty renal fossa but contralateral kidney is normal in size.[12] Ectopic renal tissue is present in the fetal pelvis, located superior to the urinary bladder (**Fig. 5**). The echogenicity is often similar to bowel but the typical renal corticomedullary differentiation helps in identification of the ectopic kidney.[14] On color Doppler ultrasonography, the renal artery can be followed to the pelvis and confirms the diagnosis.

Abnormal Fusion

The amount of liquor is normal with the most common fusion abnormality the horseshoe kidney. On imaging, the kidneys are more inferior in position than normal. The lower poles of the kidneys are medially deviated and bridge of renal tissue may be visualized anterior to the spine. An upper pole fusion is a rare variant with an inverted horseshoe morphology. A horseshoe kidney is associated with Turner syndrome, trisomy 18, and other genitourinary anomalies.[15] In cross-fused ectopia, the ectopic kidney is located anterior to the spine and is fused with the kidney in opposite flank (**Fig. 6**). There may be a large bilobed kidney. Color Doppler ultrasonography reveals two renal arteries. There is a known association with vertebral abnormalities.[12]

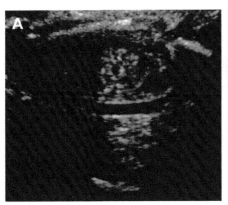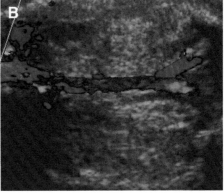

Fig. 3. (*A*) A coronal B-mode image demonstrates empty renal fossae bilaterally with a nonvisualized urinary bladder. (*B*) A coronal color Doppler image demonstrates nonvisualization of the renal arteries confirms bilateral renal agenesis.

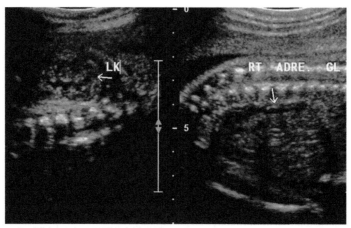

Fig. 4. A sagittal image shows absent right kidney with the typical appearance of a lying down adrenal noted in the empty renal fossa (RT ADRE. GL [*arrow*]). A single left kidney shows compensatory hypertrophy (LK [*arrow*]).

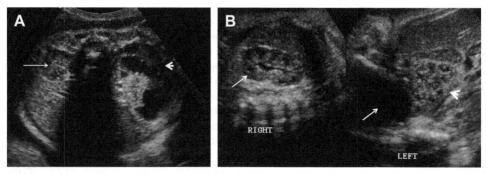

Fig. 5. (*A*) An axial image demonstrates a single kidney in right renal fossa (*arrow*) and the colon occupies the left renal fossa (*arrowhead*). (*B*) A coronal oblique image of the normally situated right kidney (*arrow*). A left ectopic kidney (*arrowhead*) is seen in the pelvis above the urinary bladder (*arrow*). Typical corticomedullary differentiation helps differentiate the kidney from the bowel.

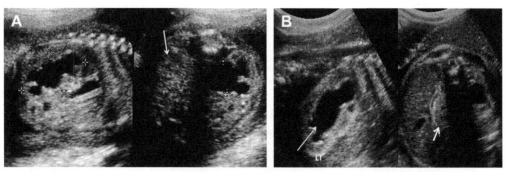

Fig. 6. (*A*) Axial and sagittal images at 20 weeks showed right empty renal fossa (*arrow*) and what was thought to be a single left kidney with PUJ obstruction (between cursors). (*B*) Follow-up image at 26 weeks confirmed the left kidney with PUJ obstruction (LT [*long arrow*]). At this stage, however, the right renal moiety was also seen (*arrow*) anterior to the spine suggesting cross-fused ectopia.

DILATATION OF THE COLLECTING SYSTEM

Dilatation of the renal pelvis is a common finding on obstetric ultrasonography. It is seen in 1% to 4% of all pregnancies. Mild pelviectasis is often a transient and idiopathic finding that resolves or remain stable.[16] It is also a minor marker for trisomy 21 and seen in association with trisomy 8 and 13 and Turner syndrome.[17] Hence, a careful survey of the fetus for other chromosomal markers is necessary and if pelviectasis is seen, a repeat examination at 4 weeks is suggested to monitor progression.[18] Diagnosis and progression of pelviectasis is monitored by measurement of the anterior posterior diameter of the renal pelvis, termed the *renal pelvis diameter* (RPD). The kidney is imaged in a transverse plane and the RPD measured. The upper limit is 3 mm in the first trimester, 4 mm during the second trimester, and 7 mm during the third trimester. Calyceal dilatation is always pathologic and sagittal and coronal views are best to image calyceal dilatation. It is important to identify those cases with a risk of developing in utero progression leading to a significant abnormality, likely to need postnatal surgical correction.[19] This may be achieved by serial follow-up measurements (**Box 2**).

There are various levels of urinary tract obstruction, at the pelviureteric junction (PUJ), lower ureter, and bladder outlet, all having typical morphologic findings that help in an accurate prenatal diagnosis.

Pelviureteric Junction Obstruction

PUJ obstruction is also termed, *congenital hydronephrosis without hydroureter or bladder dilatation*. On ultrasonography, the kidney is enlarged with a dilated renal pelvis, the hallmark finding. The distension ends abruptly at the PUJ with a blunted or bullet-nosed appearance of the renal pelvis, best imaged on coronal view. The dilated calycles appear cyst-like but communicate with the renal pelvis, best seen in a sagittal view (**Fig. 7**). The threshold measurement on a transverse image of the kidney is 7 mm for mild dilation, between 7 and 15 mm for moderate dilatation, and greater than 15 mm for severe dilatation (**Fig. 8**). The more dilated the system, the more the likelihood of decreased renal function after birth. Normally the ureters are not seen but if seen should measure less than 2 mm. In cases of unilateral PUJ obstruction, the bladder is normal; however, 10% demonstrate bilateral involvement and with severe bilateral PUJ obstruction the bladder may be small or absent.[20,21] If obstruction is severe, a rupture of a renal calyx or bladder may occur with urinary extravasation leading to a perirenal urinoma or ascites (**Fig. 9**). The functional significance of leakage is questionable; sometimes it protects the kidney and sometimes retards renal growth. There may be associated renal dysplasia with thinned hyperechoic renal cortex and cyst formation (**Fig. 10**).[22,23] In unilateral PUJ obstruction,

---

Box 2
Measurements of the neonatal kidney to indicate the need for ongoing surveillance and need for postdelivery surgical treatment

1. RPD

   >10 mm at term is significant and needs postnatal investigation
   >7 mm at 33 weeks needs follow-up
   >4 mm before 20 weeks needs follow-up

2. Renal pelvis/kidney ratio >0.28 needs postnatal investigation
3. Increasing renal size and reducing cortical thickness
4. Signs of renal dysplasia like increased cortical echogenicity and cysts
5. Complications, such as calcyeal rupture, with a fluid collection adjacent to kidney (urinoma), which may progress to urinary ascites or hydrothorax
6. Reducing amniotic fluid volume is an indicator of deteriorating renal function

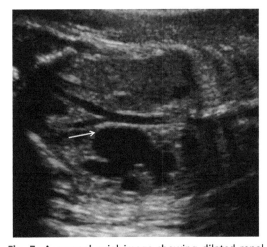

Fig. 7. A coronal axial image showing dilated renal pelvis distension, which ends abruptly at the PUJ (*arrow*) with a blunted or bullet nosed appearance of the renal pelvis, which is the hallmark finding. Dilated calyces appear cyst-like but communicate with the renal pelvis.

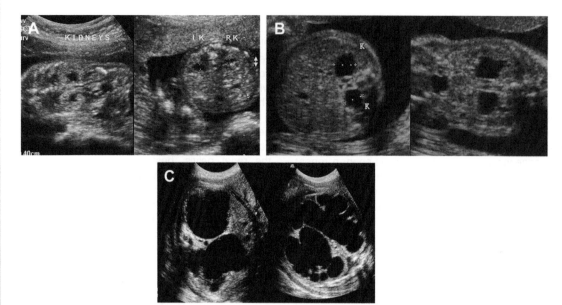

Fig. 8. Coronal and axial images for the diagnosis of hydronephrosis. Anteroposterior RPD measured on the axial images. LK, left kidney; RK, right kidney. (*A*) Mild, less than 7 mm (between cursors). (*B*) Moderate, 7 to 15 mm (between cursors). K, kidney. (*C*) Severe, greater than 15 mm (between cursors).

a contralateral renal abnormality is seen in 25% in the form of renal agenesis or renal cystic dysplasia and an extrarenal anomaly is seen in 10%. In PUJ, amniotic fluid is most often normal. Paradoxic polyhydramnios is seen in one-third due to impaired renal concentrating ability and increased urine output. If obstruction is severe and bilateral, there is oligohydramnios.

Lower Ureteric Obstruction

The establishing of lower ureteric obstruction is based on demonstration of hydronephrosis with a dilated ureter. The dilated ureter may be tortuous demonstrating peristalsis but has to be differentiated from bowel. Ureteral diameters greater than 10 mm are associated with poor prognosis and high incidence of postnatal surgical correction. It is difficult in utero to differentiate congenital megaureter from a dilated ureter caused by vesicoureteric reflux (VUR). Any variability of the diameter of the renal pelvis during one single examination favors VUR.[24] Sometimes a prominence of the ureter may be visualized during micturition (**Fig. 11**).

Duplication abnormalities are diagnosed in utero usually when there is hydronephrosis involving

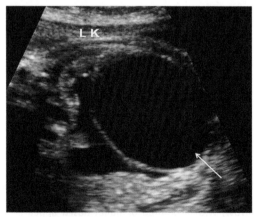

Fig. 9. Axial image in severe PUJ obstruction leading to rupture of renal calyx and a perirenal urinoma seen as an anechoic collection (*arrow*). LK, left kidney.

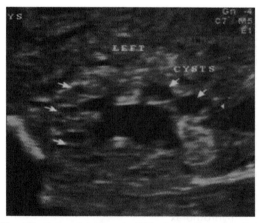

Fig. 10. Coronal image in PUJ obstruction showing renal dysplasia with hyperechoic renal cortex and associated cyst formation (*arrows*).

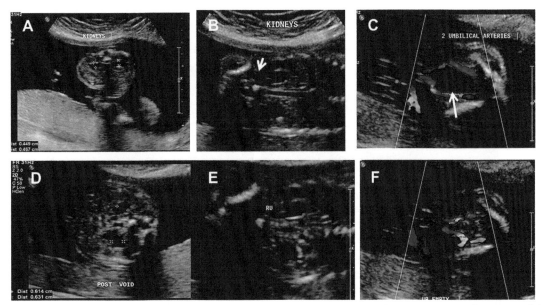

Fig. 11. Variability of the diameter of the renal pelvis and ureteral prominence during micturition favors VUR. (*A*) Bilateral dilated pelvicalyceal systems. RPD is 4 mm (between cursors). (*B*) Right ureter just seen (*arrow*). (*C*) Full bladder (*arrow*). (*D*) Increased RPD to 6 mm (between cursors). (*E*) Right ureter (RU) dilated. (*F*) Empty bladder.

the upper or lower moiety. There is asymmetry of renal sizes, the affected kidney being larger than the contralateral side.[25–28] The upper and lower pole collecting system is separated by a band of renal tissue. Two separate ureters may be visualized, which drain upper and lower poles. There is usually dilatation of upper pole collecting system, which may appear cyst-like. With severe obstruction, the upper pole parenchyma becomes thin and dysplastic and may be replaced by a large cyst that displaces the lower pole. The upper pole is drained by a dilated ureter, which may show a ureterocele, which is seen as thin-walled balloon-like structure in the bladder (**Fig. 12**). A ureterocele may be missed on an empty bladder and sometimes cause a bladder outlet obstruction.[29] The normal ureter may dilate intermittently due to VUR. Ectopic extravesical insertions of ureter are difficult to diagnose in utero. Associated gynecologic abnormalities are common and occur in 50% of women affected by renal anomalies.

Bladder Outlet Obstruction

Posterior urethral valves

The most common cause of lower tract obstruction is posterior urethral valves (PUVs) and occurs exclusively in males. Ultrasonography findings are of a bladder that is persistently distended, and a dilated posterior urethra with a typical keyhole appearance is diagnostic of PUV (**Fig. 13**). There is a variable degree of bladder distension.[30,31]

The urinary bladder may distend and fill the entire abdomen and may show wall hypertrophy (>2 mm). Sometimes the urinary bladder ruptures leading to urinary ascites, urinothorax, and peritoneal calcifications. There may be associated dilatation of the upper tract. The dilatation may be due to obstruction or due to VUR and may be unilateral or bilateral. Ultrasonography findings depend on the degree of obstruction, varying from mild pelviureteral dilatation to gross hydronephrosis. Renal cortical cysts are predictive for dysplasia and indicate irreversible renal damage. Conversely normal cortical echogenicity does not rule out dysplasia.[32,33] Unilateral dilatation often decompresses the other kidney and has a better prognosis as compared with bilateral hydronephrosis. Perinephric fluid collection or urinoma formation may be seen due to calacyceal rupture.[34] Poor prognostic factors are progressive worsening of bilateral hydronephrosis, renal dysplasia, echogenic parenchyma, cysts, fibrotic dysplastic kidney, and oligohydramnios (**Fig. 14**). With severe oligohydramnios, there is increased perinatal mortality due to pulmonary hypoplasia. Associated malformations are seen in 43%, usually cardiac and VACTERL anomalies.

Urethral atresia

Urethral atresia is a less common cause of lower tract obstruction and may be seen in both male and female fetuses. The obstruction is complete and there is anhydramnios after the first trimester

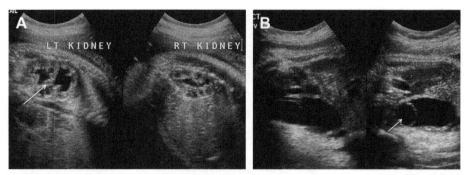

Fig. 12. (*A*) Sagittal image demonstrates left renal duplication, with the upper and lower pole collecting system separated by a band of renal tissue (*arrow*). Hydronephrosis affects the upper moiety. A normal right kidney is noted. (*B*) Coronal image demonstrates an ureterocele, seen as a thin-walled balloon-like structure within the bladder lumen (*arrow*).

with megacystis (**Fig. 15**). This is fatal due to pulmonary hypoplasia, and renal dysplasia with a few survivors has been reported after antenatal intervention.

Prune-belly syndrome

There is a lax or absent abdominal wall musculature with thin-walled large bladder and bilateral hydronephrosis and hydroureter. There is dilatation of the entire urethra with no evidence of a keyhole, indicating that PUVs are not responsible. Oligohydramnios may be present. This condition is difficult to differentiate from PUV prenatally.

Megacystis microcolon syndrome

This is more common in females. There is a thin-walled distended bladder; however, no dilated posterior urethra is present. The amniotic fluid is usually normal to increased.[35,36]

RENAL CYSTIC DISEASE
Multicystic Dysplastic Kidney

Multicystic dysplastic kidney (MDK) is the most common form of cystic renal disease seen on an antenatal sonographic examination. Unilateral involvement is seen in 80% with the left more

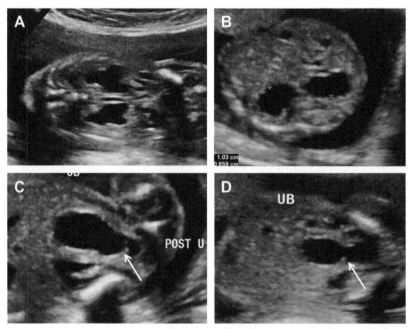

Fig. 13. (*A*) Coronal image demonstrating moderate hydronephrosis. (*B*) Axial image demonstrating moderate hydronephrosis (between cursors). (*C*) Typical keyhole appearance of a distended bladder with a dilated posterior urethra (*arrow*). (*D*) Incomplete emptying of the bladder (UB) and distension of posterior urethra during micturition (*arrow*).

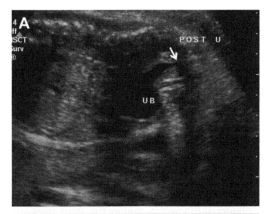

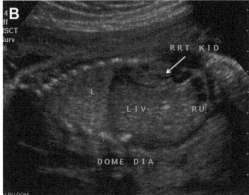

Fig. 14. (*A*) Persistently distended urinary bladder (UB) with a dilated posterior urethra (POST U [*arrow*]). (*B*) A dilated right ureter (RU) is present without pelvicalyceal system dilation due to a fibrotic dysplastic kidney (RRT KID [*arrow*]), which is smaller in size and shows increased cortical echogenicity. DOME DIA, dome of the diaphragm; L, lung; LIV, liver.

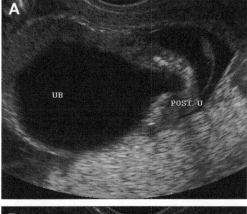

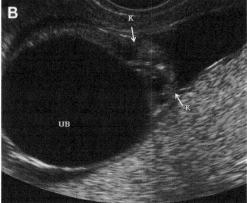

Fig. 15. (*A*) Urethral atresia with massively distended urinary bladder (UB)—megacystis. POST U, PUVs. (*B*) Back pressure in both kidneys, which show a dysplastic echogenic renal cortex. K, kidneys (*arrows*); UB, urinary bladder.

often affected than the right. The affected kidney is enlarged, the reniform shape is lost, and multiple noncommunicating cysts of varying size are seen in the renal fossa with variable amount of hyperechogenic stroma (**Fig. 16**). There is no cortex or medulla and no identifiable collecting system. These cysts may increase or decrease in size during the pregnancy. The size of the kidney often decreases in utero or after birth, with complete disappearance of MDK, mimicking renal agenesis.[37,38] Prognosis depends on the health of the contralateral kidney and a follow-up of the nonaffected kidney and amniotic fluid is suggested. Unilateral involvement carries a good prognosis; however, the contralateral kidney may be affected in 40% cases of VUR or PUJ obstruction. When MDK is unilateral and an isolated finding, there is no increased risk of chromosomal anomaly. Bilateral involvement, however, carries a poor prognosis due to

oligohydramnios and pulmonary hypoplasia (see **Fig. 16**).

Obstructive Cystic Renal Dysplasia

Obstructive cystic renal dysplasia, also termed *Potter type IV*, presents with renal macrocysts with renal obstruction (**Fig. 17**). Renal size may be increased with hydronephrosis, whereas long-standing obstruction leads to small kidneys. The kidneys maintain their reniform shape and intervening renal parenchyma is often discernible and cortical echogenecity is increased. There are renal cysts of varying sizes. Obstructive cystic renal dysplasia can result from urethral obstruction, VUJ, or PUJ. Severe obstructive cystic renal dysplasia due to early obstruction may not be distinguished from MCK.[39,40] In cases of unilateral obstructive dysplasia, the amniotic fluid is normal whereas bilateral severe involvement is associated with oligohydramnios.

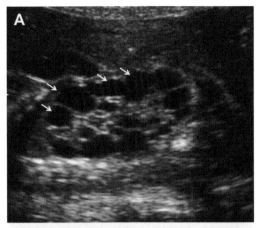

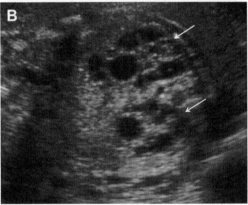

Fig. 16. (*A*) Enlarged kidney with multiple noncommunicating cysts of varying size (*arrows*) and a variable amount of hyperechogenic stroma, an MDK. (*B*) Axial image shows bilateral MDKs (*arrows*) with gross oligohydramnios.

AUTOSOMAL RECESSIVE POLYCYSTIC KIDNEY DISEASE

Autosomal recessive polycystic kidney disease (ARPKD) is also termed, *infantile polycystic kidney disease*. It is a single gene disorder resulting in bilateral, symmetric, cystic renal disease and may be associated biliary dysgenesis. The sonographic appearance varies according to the severity of involvement. The kidneys are typically markedly enlarged (+4–15 SD), hyperechoic, and without corticomedullary differentiation (**Fig. 18**). The renal enlargement may not occur until mid–second trimester and the sizes may continuously increase during the third trimester. A thin rim of hypoechoic cortex may sometimes be appreciated. Small cysts may be visible but they do not predominate. The fetal urinary bladder is not visible and there is oilgohydramnios with lung hypoplasia, which makes the prognosis poor. Limb and associated anomalies due to oligohydramnios are also common.[41–43] The second presentation of ARPKD can be reversed corticomedullary differentiation with large (+2–4 SD) kidneys. This finding is related to increase in the number of interfaces within the medullae and to inspissated material within the dilated tubules, which leads to increased echogenicity of medullae. If the amniotic fluid is preserved, these fetuses have better prognosis. The associated hepatic fibrosis is not demonstrated in utero.

When there is a history of involvement in a previous pregnancy or if parents are known carriers, the fetus should be monitored carefully with serial studies for renal size. Amniotic fluid volume is monitored and early-onset oligohydramnios suggests poor prognosis. Signs of pulmonary hypoplasia should be sought and fetal MR imaging considered.[3]

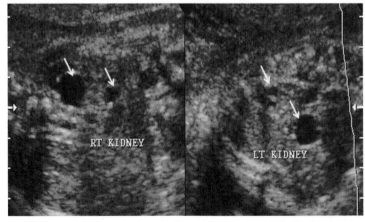

Fig. 17. Bilaterally small kidneys showing renal cysts of varying sizes (*arrows*). The intervening renal parenchyma is seen and shows increased cortical echogenicity; dysplastic changes due to a longstanding obstruction.

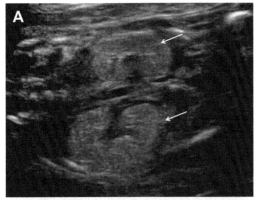

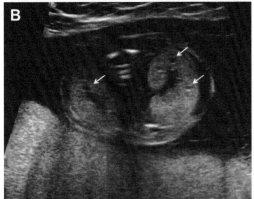

Fig. 18. (*A*) Coronal image showing markedly enlarged hyperechoic kidneys (*arrows*) without corticomedullary differentiation, characteristic of ARPKD. (*B*) Axial image showing markedly enlarged hyperechoic kidneys without corticomedullary differentiation and with small cysts (*arrows*).

AUTOSOMAL DOMINANT POLYCYSTIC KIDNEY DISEASE

Autosomal dominant polycystic kidney disease (ADPKD) is an inherited condition. In ADPKD, cysts develop only later in adulthood and in utero the kidneys have a normal appearance. A pattern highly specific for the disease in the fetus has been described, however. The kidneys are moderately enlarged (1–2 SD above the mean) possibly with hyperechoic cortices and relatively hypoechoic medullae. The hyperechoic cortex is probably related to multiple microcysts in the cortex. Another pattern corresponds to glomerulocystic variant of the disease in which the kidneys are markedly enlarged and diffusely hyperechoic (+4–8 SD) without corticomedullary differentiation. Cysts may develop in utero or after birth in the subcapsular area. The cystic renal involvement is usually asymmetric. The amniotic fluid is usually normal.[44,45]

MEDULLARY CYSTIC DYSPLASIA

In medullary cystic dysplasia, the cysts mainly involve the medullary tubules and may be associated with glomerulocystic changes as well. The kidneys are enlarged and hyperechoic with macroscopic cysts. An associated finding in utero is polydactyly and typically encountered in Meckel-Gruber syndrome.[46]

BLADDER, URETHRA, AND URACHUS

As discussed previously, the bladder is the first structure of the urinary tract to be seen in the fetal pelvis at approximately 9 to 10 weeks. Anomalies can be suspected when the urinary bladder is not visible during an examination or whenever the bladder is enlarged (>3 cm in length in second trimester or >6 cm in length in third trimester).

When the bladder is enlarged, bladder outlet obstruction should be presumed. In the first and second trimester, an enlarged bladder could result from urethral atresia and prune-belly syndrome, whereas in the second and third trimesters, in a male fetus it almost always results from PUV. In the evaluation of an enlarged bladder, marked VUR and megacystis-microcolon-hypoperstalsis syndrome should also be considered.[47–49] When the bladder is not visible, the amount of amniotic fluid helps differentiate causes secondary to a lack of urine production from those due to a bladder malformation. If there is anhydramnios or oligohydramnios, possible absent or nonfunctioning kidneys should be suspected (eg, bilateral renal agenesis or bilateral MDKs). When the amount of amniotic fluid is slightly reduced, intrauterine growth retardation or maternofetal infection should be considered. In cases of normal amniotic fluid, a bladder malformation, such as bladder extrophy, should be considered.[50]

Bladder Exstrophy

With bladder exstrophy, the urinary bladder is not visible between the umbilical arteries. Instead a soft tissue mass is seen just below the umbilicus corresponding to the open bladder mucosa. In cases when the penis is short in a male fetus, wide and ambiguous genitalia may be seen. A close differential is omphalocele-exstrophy-imperforate anus complex with an additional omphalocele component.[51,52] An abnormal bladder can also be seen in cloacal malformation with a single opening draining the bladder, vagina, and colon.[53] A fluid-filled vagina may be seen as a cystic mass varying in size between the urinary bladder and the rectum.

Patent Urachus

The urachus is normally not seen in utero because it becomes fibrotic after the first trimester. Anomalies related to urachus include patent urachus (most common), urachal cyst, diverticulum, or sinus. Urachal cysts are situated in the anterior pelvis in the midline communicating with the bladder. It may extend into the base of the umbilical cord (**Fig. 19**) and may be associated with allantoic cord cysts. These cysts resolve or rupture spontaneously at birth with few cases of needing surgical repair in the postnatal period.[54,55]

Renal tumors

The two most common renal masses reported in utero are mesoblastic nephroma and Wilms tumor. Mesoblastic nephroma is a benign mesenchymal tumor. On sonography, it appears as a solid mass, iso- to hyper-echoic compared with normal renal parenchyma. These masses may rarely have

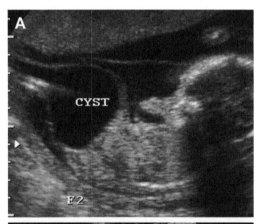

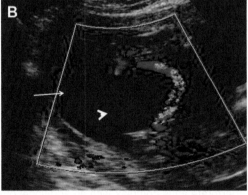

Fig. 19. (*A*) Urachal cyst (CYST), seen as a cystic mass situated in the anterior pelvis in the midline communicating with the bladder, just below the umbilicus extending into the base of the umbilical cord. (*B*) Color Doppler ultrasonography confirms two umbilical arteries flanking the bladder (*long arrow*) and urachal cyst (*arrowhead*).

a cystic area and large masses may cause increased abdominal circumference. Abdominal vessels and organs may be displaced with bowel obstruction possible. On color Doppler ultrasonography, visualization of the renal artery helps confirm a renal origin of the mass and assess vascularity of the mass. The ring sign is described as a hypoechoic ring surrounding the tumor, which is vascular on color Doppler ultrasonography. Color Doppler reveals increased vascularity in the mass and if there is significant arteriovenous shunting or venous obstruction, fetal hydrops may occur.[56–58] Severe polyhydramnios is associated in 70% of cases. A Wilms tumor has similar appearances but it is rare in utero.

Suprarenal masses

Neuroblastoma The most common suprarenal mass is a neuroblastoma. A neuroblastoma lies above the upper pole of the kidney, which is then displaced inferiorly. The mass has a variable echotexture, homogenously solid or a complex cystic with septations, rarely with calcification. Color Doppler ultrasonography demonstrates variable vascularity but does not have a single supplying vessel and this helps differentiate a neuroblastoma from an extralobar sequestration. There may be an associated hydrops or hepatic metastasis.[59–61] Even with the presence of hepatic metastasis, prognosis is excellent. MR imaging is used to confirm anatomic location and for evaluation of metastasis.

Adrenal hemorrhage Adrenal hemorrhage is seen as an enlarged echogenic mass in the suprarenal region. There is no color Doppler flow within the mass, and MR imaging confirms hematoma. Adrenal hemorrhage is known to involute over time and typical changes in morphology are seen on follow-up: solid to cystic to regression. This helps differentiate adrenal hemorrhage from a neuroblastoma.[59,62,63] Left-sided hemorrhage may be associated with ipsilateral renal vein thrombosis.

Adrenal cysts Adrenal cysts are seen as anechoic thin-walled cystic masses in the suprarenal region (**Fig. 20**). Isolated uncomplicated adrenal cysts are usually small and disappear spontaneously.[64] Large cysts are seen in association with Beckwith-Weidemann syndrome. These cysts bleed within and hence may show a variable appearance on ultrasound.[65]

Neonatal genital

Normal genitalia The use of transvaginal transducers with high-resolution capability permits early visualization of the fetal genital anatomy by

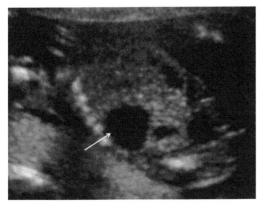

Fig. 20. An adrenal cyst is seen as a cystic mass (*arrow*) just above upper pole of the kidney on a sagittal image.

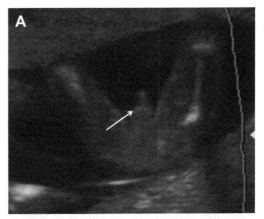

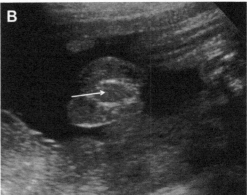

Fig. 21. (*A*) An axial image demonstrates normal male genitalia with the scrotum and penis pointing upwards (*arrow*). (*B*) The two hemiscrotum are separated by a short penis (*arrow*), the split scrotum sign; ambiguous genitalia.

the end of first trimester. The external genitalia appear identical up to 11 weeks in both genders.[66,67] The rapid growth of penis after 14 weeks allows differentiation of both genders. On sagittal scan the penis points upwards whereas the clitoris points downwards (**Fig. 21**).[68,69] The labia, scrotum, and penis become more clearly visible in the second trimester. The testes normally descend at 25 to 32 weeks. The labia are seen as 2 to 4 parallel lines. The uterus can be seen after 20 weeks as an echogenic mass between the bladder and rectum.

Male genital anomalies

Hypospadias Hypospadias is a common malformation wherein the penis appears short and broad. The tip of the penis is blunted instead of pointed and often two echogenic lines are seen at the tip. The urethra opens on the ventral aspect of the penis and not the tip. This is confirmed on color Doppler ultrasonography where an abnormal stream of urine is seen ventral to the penis, which appears fan-shaped instead of linear. Forty percent of cases are associated with other urogenital anomalies and 10% have cryptorchidism.[70–73]

Scrotal abnormalities The testis can be visualized in the scrotum at approximately 26 weeks. A small amount of fluid in the scrotal sac surrounding the testis is a normal occurrence, termed a *simple hydrocele*. With a complex hydrocele, the fluid collection appears hyperechogenic, and meconium peritonitis should be suspected. The testis in meconium peritonitis appears normal. A hydrocele may be termed, *communicating*, when fluid connects with the peritoneal cavity via a patent tunica vaginalis. In a noncommunicating hydrocele, the fluid is confined to scrotum.[70,74]

Testicular torsion The testes normally appear symmetric and show a homogenous echotexture. With acute testicular torsion, the testis and epididymis appear enlarged and appear as a single undifferentiated mass. The testis may appear hypoechoic due to edema or heterogeneous from infarction. An associated complex hydrocele with hemorrhagic fluid may be seen. Chronic testicular torsion reveals a small testis with an echogenic capsule and intraparenchymal calcification.[75–77]

Testicular tumor A testicular tumor is extremely rare in prenatal life, most common being the yolk sac tumor, which appears as a solid mass on ultrasonography. A cystic teratodermoid may be mistaken for a hydrocele.

Female genital anomalies

Ovarian cysts An ovarian cyst is the most common intra-abdominal cystic mass in the female fetus. An ovarian cyst usually results from maternofetal hormonal influence and is equivalent to an ovarian follicle. Cysts may be simple or complex in nature (**Fig. 22**). Simple cysts are usually unilocular, anechoic with occasional septations. The most common complications are torsion and hemorrhage. Cyst torsion can occur with smaller cysts but there is increased risk with size greater than 6 cm. This may be suggested by new echogenic areas within the cyst, fluid-fluid level, and septations (**Fig. 23**). Ovarian torsion may result in new fetal tachycardia. The cyst may occasionally break loose and float in the peritoneal cavity. Internal echoes within the cyst usually indicate hemorrhage secondary to torsion.[78–81] Ascites may develop as a result of cyst rupture or fluid transudation. MR imaging may be helpful to separate the cystic mass from the urinary tract. High signal within the mass on T1-weighted images confirms presence of hemorrhage or septations.

Hydrocolpos Hydrocolpos is visualized as a midline cystic mass secondary to vaginal atresia (**Fig. 24**). Demonstration of the uterine cervix at

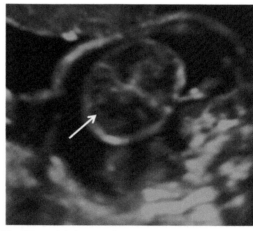

Fig. 23. Axial image demonstrates an ovarian cyst with change in morphology and new septations and internal echoes most likely due to torsion (*arrow*). Presence of ascites was noted, which regressed completely in the subsequent scans.

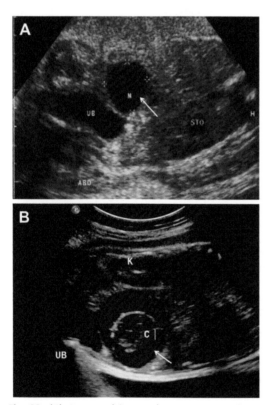

Fig. 22. (*A*) A coronal image demonstrates an intra-abdominal cystic mass (M [*arrow*]) adjacent to the urinary bladder (UB), a simple ovarian cyst. ABD, abdomen; H, heart; STO, stomach. (*B*) A coronal image demonstrates an intra-abdominal cystic mass with septations and internal echoes (C [*arrow*]) complicated ovarian cyst. K, kidney; UB, urinary bladder.

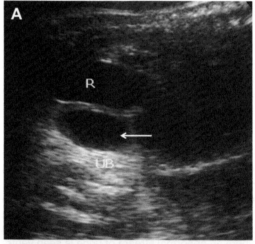

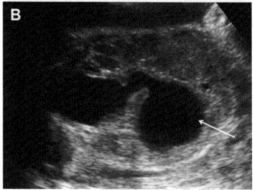

Fig. 24. (*A*) A cystic midline mass (R) behind the urinary bladder (UB [*arrow*]), suggesting hydrocolpos. (*B*) Extending cephalad from this is a pear-shaped cystic structure (*arrow*), a hydrometra.

the superior aspect of the cystic mass provides a clue to diagnosis. The condition may be part of a cloacal malformation, associated with renal agenesis/MDKs or part of the Drash syndrome.[82]

Ambiguous genitalia Ambiguous genitalia are characterized by difficulty to assign fetal gender during the second- or third-trimester sonographic examination, characterized by a failure to differentiate between a short penis and a hypertrophied clitoris. Bifid scrotum may also be misinterpreted as labia majora. Ambiguous genitalia can be a part of cloacal malformation with a common opening of the bladder, vagina, and rectum.[70] It can also be associated with adrenogenital syndrome. In a female fetus affected by adrenogenital syndrome, the clitoris is hypertrophied with presence of enlarged wrinkled adrenals. There may be associated genitourethral fistula. In boys with adrenogenital syndrome, the condition may go unrecognized unless there is hypertrophy of the adrenals.[83–85]

SUMMARY

Antenatal ultrasonography is an excellent modality that can diagnose most abnormalities of the fetal genitorurinary tract. The typical findings of various abnormalities help in accurate prenatal diagnosis. Reduced amniotic fluid is the first clue to compromised fetal renal function. With known urinary obstruction, serial follow-up ultrasonography to monitor increasing hydronephrosis and developing postobstructive dysplasia helps in obstetric and neonatal management. MR imaging gives valuable information in difficult cases, especially when there is gross oligohydramnios and poor resolution on the ultrasonography examination.

REFERENCES

1. Sadler TW, editor. Langman's medical embryology. 9th edition. Philadelphia: Lippincott, Williams and Wilkins; 2004.
2. Dillon E, Ryall A. A 10 year audit of antenatal US detection of renal disease. Br J Radiol 1998;71:497.
3. Cassart M, Massez A, Metens T, et al. Complementary role of MRI after sonography in assessing bilateral urinary tract anomalies in the fetus. AJR Am J Roentgenol. 2004;182(3):689–95.
4. Rosati P, Guaniglia L. Transvaginal assessment of fetal urinary tract in early pregnancy. Ultrasound Obstet Gynecol 1996;7:95.
5. Chamberlain PF, Manning FD, Morrison I, et al. Circadian reflux in bladder volume in the term human fetus. Obstet Gynecol 1984;64:657.
6. Cohen ML, Cooper J, Einsenberg P, et al. Normal length of fetal kidneys. AJR Am J Roentgenol 1991;157:545.
7. Lind T. The biochemistry of amniotic fluid. In: Fairweather D, Eskes T, editors. Amniotic fluid: research and clinical applications. Amsterdam: Excerpta Medica; 1978. p. 59.
8. Hoffman CK, Filly RA, Callen PW. The lying down sign: a US indicator of renal agenesis or ectopia. J Ultrasound Med 1992;11:533.
9. Bronshtein M, Amit A, Achiron R, et al. The early prenatal diagnosis of renal agenesis: technique and possible pitfalls. Prenat Diagn 1994;14:291–7.
10. Mcgahan JP, Myracle MR. Adrenal hypertrophy: possible pitfall in sonographic diagnosis of renal agenesis. J Ultrasound Med 1986;5:265–8.
11. DeVore GR. The value of color Doppler sonography in the diagnosis of renal agenesis. J Ultrasound Med 1995;14:443–9.
12. Yuksel A, Batukan C. Sonographic findings of fetuses with an empty renal fossa and normal amniotic fluid volume. Fetal Diagn Ther 2004;19:525–32.
13. Hill LM, Nowak A, Hartle R, et al. Fetal compensatory renal hypertrophy with a unilateral functioning kidney. Ultrasound Obstet Gynecol 2000;15:191–3.
14. Jeanty P, Romero R, Kepple D, et al. Prenatal diagnosis in unilateral empty renal fossa. J Ultrasound Med 1990;9:651.
15. Strauss S, Dushnitsky T, Peer A, et al. Sonographic features of horseshoe kidney: review of 34 patients. J Ultrasound Med. 2000;19:27–31.
16. Chudleigh T. Mild pyelectasis. Prenat Diagn. 2001; 21:936–41.
17. Chudleigh PM, Chitty LS, Pembrey M, et al. The association of aneuploidy and mild fetal pylectasis in an unselected population: the results of a multicenter study. Ultrasound Obstet Gynecol 2001;17:197–202.
18. Dremsek PA, Gindi K, Voitl P, et al. Renal pyelectasis in fetuses and neonates. AJR Am J Roentgenol 1997; 168:1017.
19. John U, Kahler C, Schulz SV, et al. The impact of renal pelvic diameter on postnatal outcome. Prenat Diagn 2004;24:591.
20. Anderson N, Clautice-Engle T, Allan R, et al. Detection of obstructive uropathy in the fetus: predictive value of sonographic measurements of renal pelvic diameter at various gestational ages. AJR Am J Roentgenol 1995;164:719–23.
21. De Siati M, Silvestre P, Scieri F, et al. Congenital ureteropelvic junction obstruction; definition and therapy. Arch Ital Urol Androl 2005;77:1–4.
22. Maizels M, Reisman ME, Slom LS. Grading nephroureteral dilatation detected in the first year of life: correlation with obstruction. J Urol 1992;148:609.
23. Csaicsich D, Greenbaum LA, Aufricht C. Upper urinary tract: when is obstruction obstruction? Curr Opin Urol 2004;14:213–7.

24. Elder J. Commentary: importance of antenatal diagnosis of vesicoureteral reflux. J Urol 1992;148:1750.

25. Davidovits M, Eisenstein B, Ziv N, et al. Unilateral duplicated system: comparative length and function of the kidneys. Clin Nucl Med 2004;29:99–102.

26. Whitten SM, McHoney M, Wilcox DT, et al. Accuracy of antenatal fetal ultrasound in the diagnosis of duplex kidneys. Ultrasound Obstet Gynecol 2003; 21:342–6.

27. Vergani P, Ceruti P, Locatelli A, et al. Accuracy of prenatal ultrasonographic diagnosis of duplex renal system. J Ultrasound Med 1999;18:463–7.

28. Abuhamad AZ, Horton CE Jr, Horton SH, et al. Renal duplication anomalies in the fetus; clues for prenatal diagnosis. Ultrasound Obstet Gynecol 1996;7: 174–7.

29. Kang AH, Bruner JP. Antenatal ultrasonographic development of ureteroceles. Implications for management. Fetal Diagn Ther 1998;13:157–61.

30. Eckoldt F, Heling KS, Woderich R, et al. Posterior urethral valves: prenatal diagnositic signs and outcome. Urol Int 2004;73:296–301.

31. Dinneen MD, Dhillon DK, Ward HC, et al. Antenatal diagnosis of PUV. J Urol 1993;72:364.

32. Kaefer M, Peters CA, Petik AB, et al. Increased renal echogenecity: a US sign for differentiating between obstructive and non-obstructive etiologies of in utero bladder distension. J Urol 1997;158:1026.

33. Mahony BS, Filly RA, Callen PW, et al. Fetal renal dysplasia: sonographic evaluation. Radiology 1984;152:143–6.

34. Freedman AL, Bukowski TP, Smith CA, et al. Fetal therapy for obstructive uropathy; diagnosis specific outcomes (corrected). J Urol 1996;156:720–3.

35. Carlsson SA, Hokegard KA, Mattson LA. Megacystis microcolon hypoperistalsis syndrome. Acta Obstet Scand 1992;71:645.

36. Mandell J, Lebowitz RL, Peters CA, et al. Prenatal diagnosis of megacystis megaureter association. J Urol 1992;148:1487.

37. Van Eijk L, Cohen-Overbeek TE, den Hollander NS, et al. Unilateral multipcystic dysplastic kidney; a combined pre and postnatal assessment. Ultrasound Obstet Gynecol 2002;19:180–3.

38. Mesrobian H, Rushton HG, Bulas D. Unilateral renal agenesis may result from in utero regression of multicystic renal dysplasia. J Urol 1993;150:793.

39. Nagata M, Shibata S, Shu Y. Pathogenesis of dysplastic kidney associated with with urinary tract obstruction in utero. Nephrol Dial Transplant 2002; 17(Suppl 9):37–8.

40. Poucell- Hatton S, Huang M, Bannykh S, et al. Fetal obstructive uropathy: patterns of renal pathology. Pediatr Dev Pathol 2000;3:223–31.

41. Barth RA, Guillot AP, Capeless EL, et al. Prenatal diagnosis of autosomal recessive polycystic kidney disease: variable outcome within one family. Am J Obstet Gynecol 1992;166:560.

42. Reuss A, Wladimiroff JW, Stewart PA, et al. Prenatal diagnosis by ultrasound in pregnancies at risk for autosomal recessive polycystic kidney disease. Ultrasound Med Biol 1990;16:355.

43. Wisser J, Hebisch G, Froster U, et al. Prenatal sonographic diagnosis of autosomal recessive polycystic kidney disease (ARP-KD) during the early second trimester. Prenat Diagn 1995;15:868.

44. Brun M, Maugey-Laulom B, Eurin D, et al. Prenatal sonographic patterns in autosomal dominant polycystic kidney disease: a multicenter study. Ultrasound Obstet Gynecol 2004;24:55.

45. Michaud J, Russo P, Grignore A, et al. Autosomal dominant polycystic kidney disease in the fetus. Am J Med Genet 1994;51:240.

46. Ickowicz V, Eurin D, Maugery Laulom B, et al. Meckel Gruber syndrome: sonographic pathologic correlation. Ultrasound Obstet Gynecol 2001;17:354.

47. McHugo J, Whittle M. Enlarged fetal bladders: aetiology, management and outcome. Prenat Diagn 2001;21:958.

48. Anumba DO, Scott JE, Plant ND, et al. Diagnosis and outcoome of fetal lower urinary tract obstruction in the Northern region of England. Prenat Diagn 2005;25:7.

49. Stamm E, King G, Thickman D. Megacystic-Microcolon-Intestinal hyppoperistalsis syndrome: prenatal identification in siblings. J Ultrasound Med 1991;10: 599.

50. Wilcox DT, Chitty LS. Non visualisations of the fetal bladder; aetiology and management. Prenat Diagn 2001;21:577.

51. Gearhart JP, Ben Chaim J, Jeffs RD, et al. Criteria for the prenatal diagnosis of classic bladder exstrophy. Obstet Gynecol 1995;85:961.

52. Goldstein I, Shale VE, Nisman D. The dilemma of prenatal diagnosis of bladder extrophy: a case report and review. Ultrasound Obstet Gynecol 2001;17:357.

53. Jaramillo D, Lebbowitz RL, Hendren WH. The cloacal malformation: radiological findings and imaging recommendations. Radiology 1990;177:441.

54. Anward J, Azar G, Soubra M. Sonogrpahic diagnosis of a urachal cyst in utero. Acta Obstet Gynecol Scand 1994;73:156.

55. Kilidodag EB, Kiliodag H, Bagis T, et al. large pseudocyst of the umbilical cord assocaited with patent urachus. J Obstet Gynaecol Res 2004;30:444.

56. Kelner M, Droullé P, Didier F, et al. The vascular ring sign in mesoblastic nephroma; report of two cases. Pediatr Radiol 2003;33:123–8.

57. Liu YC, Mai YL, Chang CC, et al. The presence of hydrops fetalis in a fetus with congenital mesoblastic nephroma. Prenat Diagn 1996;16:363–5.

58. Canning DA. Prenatal diagnosis of congenital mesoblastic nephroma associated with renal hypertension in a premature child. J Urol 2005; 173:983.

59. Rubenstein SC, Benacerraf BR, Retik AB, et al. Fetal suprarenal masses:sonographic appearance and differential diagnosis. Ultrasound Obstet Gynecol 1995;5:164.

60. Hosoda Y, Miyano T, Kimura K, et al. Chracteristics and management of patients with fetal neurobalstoma. J Pediatr Surg 1992;27:623.

61. Lin JN, Lin GJ, Hung IJ, et al. Prenatally detected tumor mass in the adrenal gland. J Pediatr Surg 1999;34:1620.

62. Strouse PJ, Boweman RA, Schlenizer AE. Antenatal findings of fetal adrenal hemorrhage. J Clin Ultrasound 1995;23:442.

63. Schwarzler P, Bernard JP, Senat MV, et al. Prenatal diagnosis of fetal adrenal masses: differentiation between hemorrhage and solid tumour by colour Doppler sonography. Ultrasound Obstet Gynecol 1995;5:164.

64. Morganti VJ, Anderson NG. Simple adrenal cysts in fetus, resolving in neonate. J Ultrasound Med 1991; 10:521.

65. Merrot T, Walz J, Anastasescu R, et al. Prenatally detected adrenal mass associated with Beckwith- Weidemann syndrome. Fetal Diagn Ther 2004;19:465.

66. Pinetter MG, Wax JR, Blackstone J, et al. Normal growth and development of fetal external genitalia demonstrated by sonography. J Clin Ultrasound 2003;31:465–72.

67. Shapiro E. The US appearance of normal and abnormal fetal genitalia. J Urol 1999;162:530.

68. Zalel Y, Pinhas-Hamiel O, Lipitz S, et al. The development of the fetal penis—an in ultrasonographic evaluation. Ultrasound Obstet Gynecol 2001;17:129–31.

69. Emerson DS, Felker E, Brown DL. The sagittal sign. J Ultrasound Med 1989;8:293.

70. Bronshtein M, Riechler A, Zimmer EZ. Prenatal sonographic signs of possible genital anomalies. Prenat Diagn 1995;15:215–9.

71. Cafici D, Iglesias A. Prenatal diagnosi of severe hypospadias with two- and three-dimensionsal sonography. J Ultrasound Med 2002;21:1423–6.

72. Meizner I, Mashiach R, Shalev J, et al. The tulip sign: a sonographic clue for in-utero diagnosis of severe hypospadias. Ultrasound Obstet Gynecol 2002;19: 250–3.

73. Devesa R, Muñoz A, Torrents M, et al. Prenatal diagnosis of isloated hypospadias. Prenat Diagn 1998; 18:779–88.

74. Pretorius DH, Halsted MJ, Abels W, et al. Hydroceles identified prenatally: common physiologic phenomenon? J Ultrasound Med 1998;17:49–52.

75. Herman A, Schvimer M, Tovbin J, et al. Antenatal sonographic diagnosis of testicular torsion. Ultrasound Obstet Gynecol 2002;20:522–4.

76. Youssef BA, Sammak BM, Al Shahed M. Case report. Pre-natally diagnosed testicular torsion ultrasonographic features. Clin Radiol 2000;55:150–1.

77. Devesa R, Muñoz A, Torrents M, et al. Prenatal diagnosis of testicular torsion. Ultrasound Obstet Gynecol 1998;11:286–8.

78. Quarello E, Gorincour G, Merrot T, et al. 'The daughter cyst sign': a sonographic clue to the diagnosis of fetal ovarian cyst. Ultrasound Obstet Gynecol 2003;22:433–4.

79. McEwing R, Hayward C, Furness M. Foetal cystic abdominal masses. Australas Radiol 2003;47:101–10.

80. Heling KS, Chaoui R, Kirchmair F, et al. Fetal ovarian cysts: prenatal diagnosis, management and postnatal outcome. Ultrasound Obstet Gynecol 2002; 20:47–50.

81. Meizner I, Levy A, Katz M, et al. Fetal ovarian cysts: prenatal ultrasononographic detection and postnatal evaluation and treatment. Am J Obstet Gynecol 1991;164:874–8.

82. Geipel A, Berg C, Germer U, et al. Diagnostic and therapeutic problems in a case of prenatally detected fetal hydrocolpos. Ultrasound Obstet Gynecol 2001;18:169.

83. Chekhelard A, Luton D, Philippe-Chouette P, et al. How accurate is prenatal diagnosis of abnormal genitalia. J Urol 2000;164:984.

84. Sivan E, Koch S, Reece A. US prenatal diagnosis of ambiguous genitalia. Fetal Diagn Ther 1995;10:311.

85. Mndell J, Browdey B, Pezters CA, et al. Prenatal US detection of genital malformations. J Urol 1994;153: 1995.

Index

Note: Page numbers of article titles are in **boldface** type.

Ultrasound Clin 5 (2010) 427–432
doi:10.1016/S1556-858X(10)00172-6

ultrasound.theclinics.com

Printed and bound by CPI Group (UK) Ltd, Croydon, CR0 4YY

03/10/2024

01040350-0014